D1529039

THE
MERIDIANS OF
ACUPUNCTURE

By the same author and publisher

For doctors, and for others interested in
Far Eastern philosophy and medicine. Taken
together these four books constitute a
Textbook of Acupuncture.

ACUPUNCTURE: THE ANCIENT CHINESE ART OF HEALING
THE MERIDIANS OF ACUPUNCTURE (this book)
THE TREATMENT OF DISEASE BY ACUPUNCTURE
ATLAS OF ACUPUNCTURE

For the non-medical reader, who wants a grasp of acupuncture in a few hours
ACUPUNCTURE: CURE OF MANY DISEASES

THE
MERIDIANS OF
ACUPUNCTURE

FELIX MANN

M.B., B.Chir. (Cambridge), L.M.C.C.
President of The Medical Acupuncture Society

WILLIAM HEINEMANN MEDICAL BOOKS LTD
LONDON

First published 1964
© Copyright by Felix Mann 1964

Reprinted 1971
Reprinted 1972 (twice)
Reprinted 1974

ISBN 0 433 20303 X

Printed in Great Britain by
REDWOOD BURN LIMITED
Trowbridge & Esher

CONTENTS

PREFACE IX

I. THE GENERAL FEATURES OF THE MERIDIANS 13

II. LUNG 25

III. LARGE INTESTINE 35

IV. STOMACH 41

V. SPLEEN 48

VI. HEART 54

VII. SMALL INTESTINE 61

VIII. BLADDER 66

IX. KIDNEY 73

X. CIRCULATION-SEX OR PERICARDIUM 83

XI. TRIPLE WARMER 87

XII. GALL BLADDER 95

XIII. LIVER 101

The above twelve groups are each sub-divided into:

PHYSIOLOGY

Traditional Chinese and Western Scientific Conceptions
This section includes translations from Chinese texts,
correlations with Western medicine and case histories

SYMPTOMS AND SIGNS

Symptomatology
Main Meridian Symptoms
Symptoms of Excess
Symptoms of Insufficiency
Cold, Hot, Empty, Full Symptoms
Connecting Meridian (Luo) Symptoms
Symptoms of Excess
Symptoms of Insufficiency
Muscle Meridian Symptoms

COURSE OF MERIDIANS

Course of Meridians
Main Meridian
Principal Course
Special Details
Connecting Meridian (Luo)
Muscle Meridian
Divergent Meridian, Yang and Yin
This section listed as coupled meridians under
the Yang meridian

IMPORTANT POINTS

XIV. THE EIGHT EXTRA MERIDIANS
Ren mo—Conception vessel   *110*
Du mo—Governing vessel   *111*
Chong mo—Penetrating vessel   *113*
Dai mo—Girdle vessel   *114*
Yin qiao mo—Yin heel vessel   *115*
Yang qiao mo—Yang heel vessel   *115*
Yin wei mo—Yin linking vessel   *116*
Yang wei mo—Yang linking vessel   *117*

The eight extra meridians are each sub-divided into:
Course
Function and Symptomatology
Commoner Diseases

The Governing and Conception Vessels have in addition:
Connecting Meridian (Luo)
Symptoms of Excess
Symptoms of Insufficiency

TECHNIQUE FOR USE OF EXTRA MERIDIANS *118*

NOMENCLATURE *174*

LIST OF ILLUSTRATIONS

LUNG
Main meridian 121
Connecting meridian (Luo) 122
Muscle meridian 123

LARGE INTESTINE
Main meridian 124
Connecting meridian (Luo) 125
Muscle meridian 126
Divergent meridian—Large intestine and Lung 127

STOMACH
Main meridian 128
Connecting meridian (Luo) 129
Muscle meridian 130
Divergent meridian—Stomach and Spleen 131

SPLEEN
Main meridian 132
Connecting meridian (Luo) 133
Great Luo of the Spleen 134
Muscle meridian 135

HEART
Main meridian 136
Connecting meridian (Luo) 137
Muscle meridian 138

SMALL INTESTINE
Main meridian 139
Connecting meridian (Luo) 140
Muscle meridian 141
Divergent meridian—Small intestine and Heart 142

BLADDER
Main meridian 143
Connecting meridian (Luo) 144
Muscle meridian 145
Divergent meridian—Bladder and Kidney 146

KIDNEY
Main meridian   147
Connecting meridian (Luo)   148
Muscle meridian   149

CIRCULATION-SEX
Main meridian   150
Connecting meridian (Luo)   151
Muscle meridian   152

TRIPLE WARMER
Main meridian   153
Connecting meridian (Luo)   154
Muscle meridian   155
Divergent meridian—Triple warmer and Circulation-sex   156

GALL BLADDER
Main meridian   157
Connecting meridian (Luo)   158
Muscle meridian   159
Divergent meridian—Gall bladder and Liver   160

LIVER
Main meridian   161
Connecting meridian (Luo)   162
Muscle meridian   163

EIGHT EXTRA MERIDIANS AND LUO
Ren mo—Conception vessel   164
Ren mo Luo—Conception vessel Luo   165
Du mo—Governing vessel   166
Du mo Luo—Governing vessel Luo   167
Chong mo—Penetrating vessel   168
Dai mo—Girdle vessel   169
Yin qiao mo—Yin heel vessel   170
Yang qiao mo—Yang heel vessel   171
Yin wei mo—Yin linking vessel   172
Yang wei mo—Yang linking vessel   173

PREFACE

The aim of this book is to describe in word and picture the fifty-nine meridians that constitute acupuncture. This is the first book in the Western world to do so.

Most Chinese books describe the meridians under the following five headings: **main meridian, connecting meridian, muscle meridian, divergent meridian** and **extra meridian.** Each of the five groups is sub-divided into about twelve sections for each category of meridian.

In this book I have used the reverse classification, having as main headings each of the twelve organ-meridians: lung, large intestine, stomach, spleen, heart, small intestine, bladder, kidney, pericardium, triple warmer, gall bladder, liver. Each of these twelve sections is sub-divided into four groups: main meridian, connecting meridian, muscle meridian and divergent meridian—the last being paired and described only under the Yang meridian. The extra meridians and their two connecting meridians have been retained as a separate group for reasons mentioned in the first chapter.

I have applied this system of classification as I considered the twelve main meridians of prime importance, and the five types of meridians as specialisations only. From a practical point of view this system of classification is more convenient, since a patient with cardiac disease may have symptoms along the course of the main, connecting, muscle, or divergent heart meridians. In this system, the types of diseases or symptoms which occur together may be found in the same section.

1. The first part of each section entitled 'Traditional Chinese and Western Scientific Conceptions' has been taken initially from Chinese sources which have many conceptions alien to our accustomed mode of thinking.

In an attempt to correlate all this with Western medicine, I have, after stating the traditional Chinese point of view, added a few scientific interpretations. These are mainly in terms of embryology, comparative anatomy and physiology, which I must admit is inadequate. It should be remembered that this book is one of the first attempts to link traditional Chinese and Western scientific medicine; that the whole subject is inordinately large; and that apart from my practice I have only a limited amount of time available for research and writing books. Many of the interpretations. are those of embryology and comparative anatomy, partly because these subjects interest me, partly because they give a clearer overall picture than the minutae of body chemistry, and partly because a fuller physiological explanation would require more research. I have not added a scientific explanation to those Chinese conceptions which are similar to our own in the West, for this would be superfluous: the stomach, for example, is considered to have a digestive formation in both Chinese and Western medicine.

The first section on the lung includes the sub-division into mucous, sobbing, autumn, dryness, etc. This is described more clearly in diagramatic form, on page 94 of *Acupuncture, The Ancient Chinese Art of Healing*. It has only been mentioned in this book in the one section, as this was considered all that was necessary for the practising doctor to be able to apply it to all sections.

The case histories have all been taken from my own practice. Mostly, they are typical of a large number of patients, as it has been my aim to discuss failures as well as successes, the difficult as well as the easy cases. The overall picture can be gained from the statistics in my first book.

2. The second part of each section entitled 'Symptomatology' describes the symptoms and signs of dysfunction of the organ, or the main, connecting, muscle, or divergent meridian.

The system may seem unnecessarily complicated, with even some contradictions. However, it is the Chinese system and I have left it as such.

3. The third part of each section entitled 'Course of Meridians' describes the course of the main, connecting, muscle, and divergent meridians.

4. The last part of each section entitled 'Important Points' summarises the most commonly used acupuncture points.

As will be observed from reading this book, much has been taken from Chinese sources. These have been acknowledged in the Bibliographies of my other two books. Amongst these the main sources have been:

ZHONGYIXUE GAILUN (A Summary of Chinese Medicine);

compiled by the Nanking Academy of Chinese medicine; published by the Peoples' Hygiene Publishing House, Peking, 1959.

ZHENJIUXUE JIANGYI (Lectures in Acupuncture and Moxibustion); compiled by the Acupuncture Research Section of the Shanghai Academy of Chinese Medicine; published by the Shanghai Scientific and Technical Publishing House, Shanghai, 1960.

For the Chinese sections I thank my teachers of the Chinese language, D. T. Owen, B.A., and F. K. Liu, B.Sc.(Hon.), M.Sc., without whose efforts neither my knowledge of Chinese nor these translations would exist.

It has been difficult to balance between a literal translation of the Chinese, which would retain most of the original meaning, but make difficult reading, and a freer translation in better English, which would lose some of the original meaning, but be easier to read.

Mr and Mrs G. Griffith-Jones have tried to make the reading of this book clearer and easier without destroying too much of the original meaning.

Frederick Metcalf, F.R.S.A., has made the drawings.

Dr Humphrey Greenwood, Head of the Fish Department of the Natural History Museum, London, has helped me in ichthological matters.

Most of the sections on physiology and embryology are taken from what I learnt as a medical student at Cambridge. As a ready reference I have used: Synopsis of Physiology by Vass, Short and Pratt; and Developmental Anatomy by Arey.

If any reader of this book can think of more correlations between the ideas of Traditional Chinese Medicine and Western Scientific Medicine, I would be glad to hear of them. If appropriate they will be included in further editions of this work. These correlations could be in terms of clinical practice, physiology, embryology, anatomy, comparative anatomy, biochemistry, etc.

Doctors or medical students who wish to study acupuncture are welcome to come to the courses which I give. These courses concentrate on the practical aspects of acupuncture, being somewhat similar to ward rounds at medical school.

With the publication of this, my fourth work on acupuncture (three books and an atlas), there now exists a more or less complete textbook on acupuncture in English, though one could always add much more.

I would also like to thank the Chinese Medical Association and the many doctors of Peking, Nanking and Shanghai for their hospitality whilst I was in China. Their untiring efforts in answering all my questions and in showing me their special techniques has been of inestimable value.

LONDON, W.1. 1964   FELIX MANN

CHAPTER I

THE GENERAL FEATURES
OF THE MERIDIANS

Recognition of what are called the 'meridians' of the human body
is one of the fundamentals of the theory and practice of acupuncture,
the form of medical treatment originally developed in ancient
China, but now gradually finding a respected place in Western
medicine. The meridians need to be conceived as the paths of
circulation and influence of certain forms of essential energy (called
in Chinese Qi) in the body. This flow of essential energy, Qi, along
the meridians, might in reality be a wave of electrical depolarisation
travelling along a fibre of the autonomic nervous system: the Qi
being the electrical phenomenon, the meridian the fibre of the
autonomic nervous system. In this book I will adhere to the traditional Chinese description as without it the Chinese conception of
disease cannot be understood.

For the purposes of general exposition, the meridians can be best
regarded as a communications system, a system consisting basically of
meridian complexes, each being associated with a particular physiological unit of the body, the units being the twelve basic organs
distinguished as such in Chinese medicine, *i.e.*, the lungs, the large
intestine, the stomach, the spleen, the heart, the small intestine,
the bladder, the kidneys, the pericardium, the triple warmer,
the gall bladder and the liver.

The Chinese normally speak of the meridians in pairs and they
distinguish the members of each pair by reference to the arm or leg,
thus indicating the main location of the particular meridian instead
of the particular organ to which it is related:

Sunlight Yang $\begin{cases} \text{arm—large intestine} \\ \text{leg—stomach} \end{cases}$

Lesser Yang $\begin{cases} \text{arm—triple warmer} \\ \text{leg—gall bladder} \end{cases}$

Greater Yang $\begin{cases} \text{arm—small intestine} \\ \text{leg—bladder} \end{cases}$

Greater Yin $\begin{cases} \text{arm—lung} \\ \text{leg—spleen} \end{cases}$

Absolute Yin $\begin{cases} \text{arm—pericardium (circulation-sex)} \\ \text{leg—liver} \end{cases}$

Lesser Yin $\begin{cases} \text{arm—heart} \\ \text{leg—kidney} \end{cases}$

Thus the small intestine meridian is referred to by the Chinese as the Arm Greater Yang, and the bladder meridian as the Leg Greater Yang. Used on its own the term Greater Yang would refer to the two meridians jointly.

The twelve main meridians are traditionally arranged in a certain order, following the sequence in which Qi flows from one meridian to another, and also following the sequence of the times of maximum and minimum activity of the meridians and organs.* Thus arranged the two ways of naming meridians become more obvious to the reader.

The Greater Yang (small intestine and bladder) is not coupled with the Greater Yin (lung and spleen) as might be expected but with the Lesser Yin (heart and kidney). The small intestine and heart on the one hand, and the bladder and the kidney on the other hand, are coupled meridians (Sovereign Fire and Water).

The Chinese system of identification moreover indicates that there are functional relationships between the meridians in each pair, and clinical experience shows that these organs or meridians are in fact related to one another. For instance, the kidney (foot Lesser Yin meridian) and heart (arm Lesser Yin meridian) sometimes have a reciprocal effect: in cardiac failure there is often oliguria; in renal failure there is not infrequently secondary cardiac failure.

The relationships between one organ and another should not however be taken as fixed and invariable features of the system. The laws and relationships of the meridians merely illustrate the possibilities that one organ or meridian has of exerting an effect on its fellows. There are, as it were, only certain routes whereby one

*For details see: *Acupuncture: The Ancient Chinese Art of Healing.*

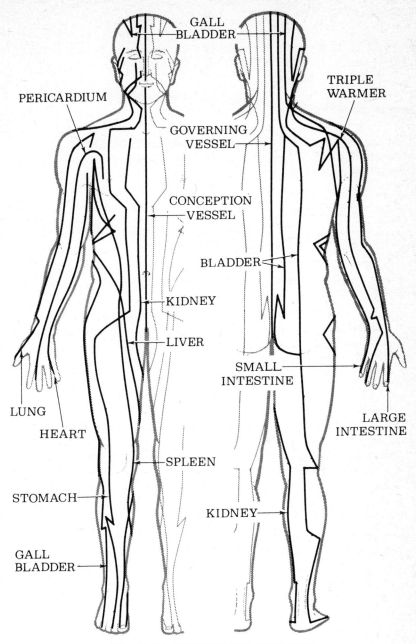

GALL BLADDER

TRIPLE WARMER

PERICARDIUM

GOVERNING VESSEL

CONCEPTION VESSEL

BLADDER

KIDNEY

LIVER

SMALL INTESTINE

LUNG

HEART

LARGE INTESTINE

STOMACH

SPLEEN

KIDNEY

GALL BLADDER

THE 12 OR 14 IMPORTANT MERIDIANS

organ can affect another, these routes being formulated into laws. Some of these routes are more direct than others, so that whereas there are many possibilities, only certain of them occur at all frequently in practice.

The implication is merely that, if a patient has say a cardiac disease, one should keep one's eyes open for any renal complications. There are of course other possibilities, for if the patient has primarily a cardiac disease it may have an effect on the gall bladder via the law of mid-day and midnight, or on the small intestine for the heart and small intestine are coupled organs, or on the spleen via the superficial circulation of energy, and the spleen may likewise be affected in a primary disease cardiac disease via the law of the five elements.

Classification of Meridians

The twelve meridian complexes described broadly in the foregoing paragraphs comprise complexes of different types of meridians and these are classified traditionally as follows:

Main meridians (of which there are twelve)
Branch meridians (of varying number with each main meridian)
Connecting meridians—Luo—(of which there are fifteen)
Muscle meridians (of which there are twelve)
Divergent meridians (of which there are twelve)
Extra meridians (of which there are eight)

The whole series of meridian complexes permeates both the surface and the interior of the body and forms what is called in Chinese 'the meridian network'.

In practice and when used by itself, the term 'meridian' usually denotes either the meridians in general, or simply the main meridians. These are by far the most important, and their influence can be regarded as in the nature of a common denominator of the associated other types of meridians.

The courses of the main meridians are located on the surface of the body by reference to a series of acupuncture points. Apart from two meridians known as the Conception Vessel and Governing Vessel, which are described later, the main meridians are the only ones which have their own acupuncture points; the other·categories of meridians are influenced indirectly through the points on the main meridians.

In both Chinese and European charts of acupuncture points and meridians, each meridian normally is represented as a line joining consecutive numbers of the same meridian. For example, one section of the meridian of the spleen joins points Spleen 13 to Spleen 14. According to the Chinese, however, the spleen meridian makes a deviation at this point and goes from Spleen 13 to Conception Vessel 2, then on to Conception Vessel 3, and only then finally on to Spleen 14. In my 'Anatomical Charts of Acupuncture Points, Meridians and Extra Meridians',* only the direct course of the main meridians is shown. In this present book, the deviations of the main meridian from the direct meridian are shown both in the text and in the drawings. In the text of this book the differences between the direct route and the devious route connecting with points on other meridians can be discerned, as the direct course consists of only the consecutive numbers on the same meridian. In the drawings at the back of this book the deviations to other meridians have been shown by both *lettering and numbering* the points on the other meridians, while the meridian under discussion has only a *number* (in heavy type) at a few of its representative points.

In addition, the main meridians have branches (which, as the deviations, are also not shown on my acupuncture charts) but are shown in the drawings at the back of this book as a dotted line. Most but not all of these branches go to acupuncture points on other meridians and these points, like those of the deviations, are lettered in addition to being numbered.

Before going on to describe the functions of each of the twelve meridian complexes in the succeeding chapters, it is appropriate to outline the chief characteristics of each of the particular types of meridians of which the complexes are composed, and to mention a number of features relevant to practical application. The remaining sections of this chapter are devoted to this purpose and, at this point, I should mention the following. This is that, in describing both the functions and the positions of the meridians in this book, I have more or less adhered to the classical tradition. In practice, however, I have not infrequently noticed that the sphere of influence of the meridians is not entirely consistent with the traditional view. The anatomical differences also imply that there are many more branch meridians than those described, some of them being of con-

*Also published by William Heinemann Medical Books Ltd. Republished now as Atlas of Acupuncture.

siderable clinical importance. When I have been able to systematise them, the physiological and anatomical differences will be described in later editions of this book.

THE MERIDIAN COMPLEX

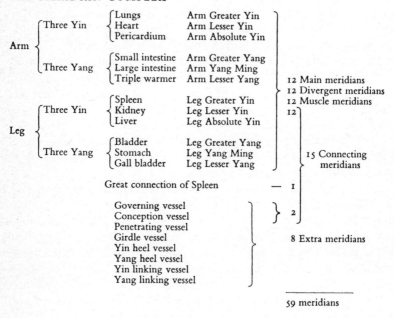

The Main Meridians

The main meridians permeate the body by the following two methods:

a. The Yang meridians control the exterior of the body, the Yin meridians the interior. The exterior and interior meridians are paired with one another as coupled meridians. For example, the large intestine (Yang meridian) with the lung (Yin meridian).

The Fu (Yang organ) and the Zang (Yin organ) are supposed to have a direct connection. The meridians also are connected with one another, this taking place at the tips of the fingers and toes. For example, the lung and large intestine meridians are connected between the thumb and index finger; likewise the stomach and spleen meridians are connected between the second toe and the big toe.

b. There is a connection between arm meridians and leg meridians. This occurs in two places: one is on the head, where the arm Yang meet the leg Yang, and the other on the front of the chest, where the arm Yin meet the leg Yin meridians.

The main meridians run both up and down the limbs, and the Qi flows from one meridian into the next in succession, until the whole circuit is completed, thereafter flowing into the first one again. In half of the main meridians (*i.e.*, the three upper Yang and three lower Yin meridians) the flow is centripetal; in the others it is centrifugal.

The Connecting Meridians (or Luo)

Each of the twelve main meridians has a Luo point and an associated Luo meridian. The functions of the latter are to connect with coupled meridians.

One part of the Luo meridian is connected to the coupled meridian, running from the Luo point of the one meridian to the Luo point of the coupled meridian. For example, Lung 7 is connected to Large Intestine 6. This part of the Luo meridian is always below the elbow or knee.

The other part, which most have, roughly follows the course of the main meridian for a short distance, and controls the part of the body that it traverses.

The Luo meridian of the Governing Vessel connects with the Vessel of Conception and the kidney meridian. The Luo meridian of the Vessel of Conception connects with the Chong mo. The spleen has the so-called Great Luo, which connects with all the other 14 Yin and Yang Luo.

The connecting (Luo) meridians are supposed to run a superficial course through the body. Some authorities have said that it is possible to see whether the Luo are full or empty, but this idea may have arisen amongst the early acupuncturists through confusing the Luo with veins, for veins can easily be seen when they are full of blood and disappear when there is little blood in them.

As these meridians run on the whole superficially, and have a relatively short course with few inter-connections, their symptomatology relates mainly to the surface of the body and not so much with the severer and more complicated diseases of the internal abdominal organs.

The Muscle Meridians

The muscle meridians, as their name implies, run superficially along the surface of the muscles; they pass from joint to joint. The diseases which they influence are mainly those affecting the surface of the body, such as muscular rheumatism and the neuralgias.

The muscle meridians do not have any connections with the internal organs and thus do not influence internal diseases. There is moreover no reciprocal interior and exterior relationship amongst the muscle meridians.

The muscle meridians start at the extremities of the limbs, thence running centripetally with a meeting point at most major joints en route, and terminating on the abdomen, thorax or head. The leg 3 Yang muscle meridians unite on the cheek; the leg 3 Yin muscle meridians unite at the genitalia; the arm 3 Yang muscle meridians unite at the side of the head; the arm 3 Yin muscle meridians unite on the chest.

This purely centripetal course is different from that of the main meridians.

The Divergent Meridians

The divergent meridians usually leave their parent meridian above the knee or elbow, thereafter traversing the interior of the body and connecting with the coupled interior organ. For instance, the bladder divergent meridian is connected to the kidney. Most of the divergent meridians then emerge at the neck. The Yang divergent meridians join their parent main meridian and then continue their course as the main meridian. The Yin divergent meridians likewise link up with the coupled Yang meridian. For example, the divergent meridians of the bladder and kidney meridian both join the bladder main meridian at the back of the neck, their subsequent course being continued only by the main bladder meridian.

From this it may be seen that the divergent meridians connect the internal Zang and Fu and also that coupled divergent meridians are closely inter-twined. The flow of Qi along all divergent meridians is cephalad, as opposed to that of the main meridians.

The divergent meridians enable the Yin main meridians to have an effect on the head, for all of the arm or leg main Yin meridians stop short on the chest, and none reaches the head directly. For example, although it does not reach the head the kidney divergent meridian has an effect on the head because it joins the bladder main meridian at the nape of the neck, thus enabling the bladder main meridian to transmit any effect of stimulating the kidney meridian.

The Extra Meridians

Six of the eight extra meridians, or 'strange meridians' as they are called in Chinese, have no acupuncture points of their own. They use the acupuncture points of the twelve main meridians. They do not have a circulation of energy. The exceptions are the Governing Vessel and Conception Vessel, which not only have their own acupuncture points but also have their own circulation of energy.

The eight extra meridians have no reciprocal connections between the solid and hollow organs, or the interior and surface of the body. Their function is supposed to be like that of a lake, regulating the excess or deficiency of water in the rivers—the main meridians.

Practical Application

The Meridian Complex

Traditionally the various types of meridians are described as being separate entities: the muscle meridians having a certain function, the connecting meridians (Luo) another function, etc., etc. For practical purposes, however, I do not think there is much difference between the various types.

If, for example, a patient has a symptom which is at least partially localised over the cheek, this might suggest a dysfunction of the bladder muscle meridian, which unites there. If pulse diagnosis and other symptoms or signs also indicate a dysfunction of the bladder, the diagnosis is confirmed, and the disease may be treated via acupuncture points on the bladder main meridian (or points on other meridians which have an indirect effect on the bladder).

The above example shows that the specialised types of meridians extend the range of activity of the main meridians. In my view it is best to regard the specialised types as an extension of the main meridian bearing the name of the same organ. For example, the use of an acupuncture point on the gall bladder main meridian has its field of activity extended to the connecting, muscle, divergent and branch meridians of the gall bladder. In reverse, a symptom along or near any of the above specialised meridians indicates a disturbance of the gall bladder—in the Chinese sense.

Many parts of the body are not near any particular one of twelve main meridians, but if these are taken together with all the other meridians (a total of 59), practically every part of the body is covered.

The Vessel of Conception and Governing Vessel could be counted as a special addition, for they have their own acupuncture points, thus making a total of fourteen important meridians. The other six extra meridians do not seem to fit in with the above classification. It is possible that they channel the influences of particular points, such as K3, which have a large sphere of activity. Alternatively they may act as communications between various meridians, and would therefore be classified under the meridian to which they have the greatest affinity, *e.g.*, the Dai mo as part of the gall bladder complex.

In many parts of the body, several meridians each belonging to a different member of the main twelve run over the same region of the body. Where this occurs, detection of the offending meridian entails not only noting the pulse diagnosis, the symptoms and signs, but also a knowledge of the principles of physiology and pathology. In every such instance all the above factors must be considered, the relation of the meridians to the diseased area being but one of the many factors. These often contradict one another and need to be weighed in the light of clinical experience.

The Organ Affects the Meridian and the Meridian Affects the Organ

The meridians are, as it were, the threads that link the various phenomena observable in acunpuncture, both in diagnosis and in treatment.

A patient may have a disease of the heart, and amongst other things this is usually accompanied by pain down the inside of the arm roughly following the course of the meridian of the heart. There may also be pain going up the throat to the eye, or over the chest to the middle of the abdomen, these pains following the course of the branches of the main heart meridian or of the muscle or connecting or divergent heart meridian. If an acupuncture point on the heart meridian is stimulated in this type of case, the disease of the heart (provided it is the type of cardiac disease that may be treated by acupuncture) will be cured, or at least ameliorated.

A reverse order of events may occur in a patient who has, say, a Colles fracture at the wrist, which has happened in such a way that there is a particularly tender place over the meridian of the heart. In such a case the patient, who previously had no cardiac symptoms, may suddenly develop palpitations or have a feeling of constriction in the chest, or dyspnoea on exertion. (This will not happen in the majority of Colles fractures; it will only happen in those with the point of maximum tenderness over the heart meridian.) This patient too may be cured by stimulating an acupuncture point on the meridian of the heart, using the meridian either on both sides, or on the same side as the injury, or preferably only the opposite side.

Thus a disease or dysfunction of the heart may cause symptoms along one or other of the meridians belonging to the heart complex; and in reverse, something that irritates a certain point on the heart meridian may give rise to cardiac symptoms or even disease. In either type of case, whether the disease originated in the heart or by irritation of the heart meridian, the dysfunction may be corrected by stimulating acupuncture points on the meridian of the heart.

This is one of the special advantages of acupuncture, for it enables diagnosis and treatment to be so closely allied that they are practically one and the same thing, *i.e.*, if you have made a diagnosis, you more or less automatically know the treatment. Similarly, and in reverse, if you are not sure of the diagnosis, and try a certain treatment which then works, you automatically know the diagnosis.

The Meridians and Cellular Pathology

Western medicine is based on the ideas of cellular pathology as first expounded by Virchow. In this one distinguishes as minutely as possible the type of tissue that is diseased, whether it be muscle, bone, blood vessel, nerve, etc., even which type of cell in that tissue is diseased, and more recently the intra-cellular changes that take place in the diseased cell.

In acupuncture the reverse to the ideas of cellular pathology often seems to apply. If, for example, someone has an insect bite on the elbow, this is best treated in acupuncture by stimulating the meridian which runs over that part of the elbow. If, for example, it was in the region of the lateral epicondyle of the humerus, the large intestine meridian would be treated, preferably on the opposite side. If, instead of having an insect bite on the elbow, that same patient had muscular rheumatism, a painful wound, early arthritis, epicondylitis, a localised skin disease or any other disease involving any of the cellular elements in that region of the body, the treatment would be exactly the same, namely by treating the meridian of the large intestine on the opposite side.

From this it may be seen that the cellular pathology does not necessarily dictate any difference in treatment by acupuncture.

It would therefore seem that the meridians are the controlling factor in the various regions of the body, and that they control the body more in a regional way, irrespective of what type of tissue or cell may be there. In addition to having this regional effect the meridians have an effect on the whole body, and this appears to operate via the mediation of the internal organs with which the meridians are connected.

A knowledge of histology and cellular pathology is nevertheless important in acupuncture in a more general way, in helping to decide which disease can or cannot be treated. For instance, a duodenal ulcer may be treated successfully, as the cells lining the duodenum are of a type which regenerate easily. Diseases of the nervous system can be treated only to a limited extent, for the neurones of the brain and spinal cord do not regenerate.

CHAPTER II

LUNGS

Traditional Chinese and Western Scientific Conceptions

The Lungs Control Qı

'The lungs control Qi.' This has two meanings, for Qi in Chinese means both energy and breath, much as the Prana of the Hindus.

The Jing Qi of 'liquid and solid food', which is produced as the result of digestion in the stomach and upper digestive tract, passes first to the lungs, where it combines with the Qi of the air, and thus the true Qi of the human being is formed. This is also called the upright Qi of health, as opposed to the evil Qi of disease.

'*True Qi is that which is received from Heaven, combined with the Qi of nourishment. It fills the whole body.*'

(Ling Shu, zijie zhenxie lun)

'*Man's breathing connects the Jing Qi of Heaven and Earth in order to form the true Qi of the body.*'

(Zangshi, leijing)

A deficiency of Qi results, therefore, amongst other things in a general fatigue of the body and also air-hunger. As far as the respiratory function is concerned, J. Barcroft writes: 'Acute anoxia simulates drunkness, chronic anoxia simulates fatigue.'

The Lungs and Heart

The Chinese call the lungs the Complementary Official, recognising an association in function between the lungs and the heart. This is something that is well known by clinical experience and can also be explained by the theories of Western medicine. It may be seen in the dyspnoea caused by cardiac failure, or the tachycardia caused by pulmonary insufficiency.

From the Chinese point of view, the lungs control Qi, while the heart controls Blood.

'*Qi is the commander of the Blood: if Qi moves, then Blood moves. Blood is the mother of Qi: if Blood reaches a place, then Qi also reaches it.*'

There is even an embryological relationship between the heart and the lungs in-so-far as the one makes room for the development of the other: the heart being mainly on the left where there are two lobes of the lung, while the right side on which the heart encroaches to a lesser extent has three lobes. What would be the third bronchus on the left side (equivalent to the right apical bronchus) is only vestigal and fails to induce the formation of a separate lobe from the surrounding mesenchyme, supposedly because of the relative caudal recession of the aortic arch or the rotation of the heart. The space not taken up by the heart (and pulmonary vein) on the right, is partially filled by the cardiac lobe, which is a branch of the lower lobe, and only appears on the right.

The chemoreceptors of the carotid bodies (IX cranial nerve) and the aortic body (X cranial nerve) respond to a decrease in the concentration of oxygen or an increase in the concentration of carbon dioxide, both largely dependent on pulmonary function. Via this reflex the sino-auricular node is affected, thus altering the rate of the heart. In this case the interaction of the lungs and heart is not direct, but indirect via the gases (largely dependent on pulmonary function) dissolved in the arterial blood on the one hand, and the carotid and aortic bodies associated with the heart on the other.

As is well known, the inspired air and the blood are in intimate contact in the alveolar sacs, being separated from one another by a membrane only one cell thick, usually consisting of nothing but capillary endothelium.

Not infrequently dysfunction of the lung and heart affects the external configuration, as may be seen in the person who has a long narrow flat chest, with dyspnoea and palpitations on slight exertion. In this type of patient pulse diagnosis shows that both the lung and the heart are under-active.

Case History. A girl of twelve was seen with extreme fatigue; wishing to go to bed at 6 p.m. and unable to concentrate well at school. On slight exertion she became breathless with occasional retrosternal pain. She had ulcers on the tip and sides of her tongue—see section on heart for explanation of this last symptom. Her chest was long, narrow and flat.

Pulse diagnosis showed an underactivity of both lung and heart. She was cured after four treatments at L9 and H7.

The Lungs, Skin and Hair

The lungs are related to the skin and the body hair for Qi controls the exterior of the body, while Blood controls the interior.

Normally in cold weather the pores of the skin close and perspiration ceases, while in warm weather the pores open and there is perspiration.

If there is a deficiency of lung Qi, this impairs the ability of the skin to adapt itself to change in external circumstances, such as cold and heat, dryness and damp, so that colds, influenza or pneumonia are more easily contracted. In severe cases, the patient will suffer from spontaneous sweating, or sweating from the slightest exertion.

If on the other hand there is an excess of lung Qi, so that the exterior, i.e., the skin, is over full, the patient may easily contract diseases of the lungs, with coughing and dyspnoea, but with a sweatless fever. If drugs or acupuncture are used to cause perspiration, the breathing will become normal and the fever will subside.

The Chinese conception of an association of the lungs and skin was well known in European mediaeval medicine. In many animals the skin performs an important respiratory function:

The loach, Misgurnus, excretes up to 92% of its carbon dioxide through the skin. In the loach, 63% of the oxygen is obtained through the skin, and 37% through the gills. If the gills are occluded (by tying the pharynx and gills) the consumption of oxygen through the skin increases to 85%. The remainder is obtained through the intestine.*

The eel, Anguilla, and the mud-skipper, Periophthalmus, use the skin to absorb oxygen. The frog breathes both through its lungs and through its skin, the main pulmonary artery being divided into two branches, one going to the lung, the other to the skin, i.e., the vascularisation of the skin belongs to the pulmonary circulation.

Pulmonary diseases may often be recognised by the texture or colour of the skin: the dry flaking skin of certain asthmatics or the discolouration of the skin in negroes with tuberculosis (E. Cochrane).

Case History. A patient was seen with asthma and a dry scaling skin. He had the dry skin from childhood, while the asthma was of more recent onset.

Pulse diagnosis showed a weak pulse of the lung. The lungs were treated by acupuncture which quickly cured the asthma. The skin responded more slowly, improving, though not being completely cured.

The Lungs Open the Nostrils

The nose is part of the respiratory system, and as such is associated with the lungs.

*G. V. Nikolsky. The Ecology of Fishes. Academic Press.

'Lung Qi penetrates to the nose; if the lungs are harmonious, then the nose is able to distinguish odours.'

(Ling Shu, modu pian)

Thus, when the lung Qi is invaded by wind and cold, there may be the symptoms of a clear nasal discharge and anosmia. If in addition it is affected by heat, the discharge will become purulent. If the lung is excessively hot, and this cannot be dissipated, this results in coughing, dyspnoea and anxious breathing, there may be irritation of the nose, and movement of the alar nasae.

Embryologically, the nose is only secondarily adapted to the respiratory system, being originally the mouth—the cephalic end of the primitive gut.

Case History. A patient was seen at the very beginning of a cold, with sneezing and a clear nasal discharge. The associated point of the lungs, B13, was stimulated, which cured all symptoms within a few minutes. (This particular technique is only occasionally effective in the earliest stages of the common cold.)

The Lungs, Trachea and Larynx

The larynx being part of the respiratory system, it follows that timbre of the voice reflects the state of the true Qi of the body.

Not infrequently, the timbre of the voice is affected by other organs which have a direct or indirect effect on the lung, which in turn affects the larynx. In addition, the three lower Yang meridians pass through the neck alongside the larynx on their way to the feet, and can thus influence speech.

That part of the larynx which is below the vocal cords is formed in the embryo from the lung bud; while the part above the vocal cords is formed from the pharynx. From this point of view one would expect the lower part of the larynx to respond to the lung meridian and the upper part to respond to the stomach meridian.

Case History. A patient had a weak voice, a slightly breathless manner of speech and looked as if he could easily be blown over by the slightest breath of wind.

Pulse diagnosis showed an underactive lung. Stimulation of the lung meridian, S9 locally, and Cv17 the alarm point of the lung, cured the condition.

The Lungs in Relation to Anguish and Claustrophobia

From the psycho-somatic point of view, the mind can affect the body and the body the mind. Certain mental diseases cause or are caused by a dysfunction of the lungs.

The type of mild fear and anguish, which one may experience when holding one's breath, is a lung symptom.

Case History. A patient was suffering from a mixture of anguish, fear and depression for no obvious reason, *i.e.,* there was no external cause. I therefore assumed the mental state was the result of an internal dysfunction. I tried various treatments without success. Then, going over the history again more thoroughly, I found that the patient disliked small rooms, a condition amounting to a mild claustrophobia. The lung was stimulated at L8 and within minutes the patient felt better and was cured with a further three treatments.

Case History. Over a period of a few weeks a patient developed an extreme dislike of crowds, particularly parties held in small over-crowded rooms, something which she had adored before. She thought she was going mad, even though she did not feel mad. A psychiatrist was consulted to no avail. A chance chest X-ray at a mass radiography unit showed pulmonary tuberculosis. Chemotherapy cured the tuberculosis and the mental symptoms.

The above two histories show that apart from an anguish-fear complex, claustrophobia is also a lung symptom. Claustrophobia, being only the mental counterpart of physical air hunger, can be successfully treated in this way in a certain proportion of patients. It should not be forgotten though that all symptoms or diseases, though seeming identical, may have different causes and therefore require an entirely different treatment.

Mucous

Mucous being the secretion of the lungs, is dependent on them. Sometimes the spleen (the lung and spleen are greater Yin organs) is more effective in the treatment of the viscid mucous of the asthmatic.

Sobbing

Sobbing, in which one's respiration becomes violent and jerking (not just crying), is a pulmonary symptom.

Autumn

Autumn is the season when the lungs are most easily affected.

Dryness

Dryness frequently makes lung diseases worse. A steam kettle in the room of children with pneumonia and bronchitis, may assist recovery. Occasionally dryness is beneficial.

White

A white discolouration of a particular quality, especially of the face, may be a pulmonary symptom.

The Lungs, Kidney and Bladder

'*The lungs give life to the skin, which in its turn nourishes the kidney.*'

The lungs excrete 500 cc of water, as vapour in the expired air, under average conditions in a day. Under similar conditions the skin loses about 1,000 cc as perspiration.

Some types of oedema may be cured by treating the lungs. I have not as yet been able to clearly define this group however.

Case History. For over ten years, a patient had a skin disease with marked hyperkeratosis, especially of the wrists and ankles. He was unable to perspire however hot he became.

Pulse diagnosis showed an underactivity of the lungs and kidneys. These were stimulated at L9 and K5. Two weeks later he suddenly woke up in the middle of the night, bathed in perspiration so that he had to change his pyjamas and sheets. This excessive perspiration, which was accompanied by a desquamation of the hyperkeratotic areas, continued for three months, thereafter dying down to normal.

Heat Loss

Heat loss takes place largely via the skin.

The skin loses 87.5% by evaporation, radiation and conduction. 7% is lost by evaporation from the lungs. Warming the expired air accounts for 3.5%. 2% is lost via the urine and faeces. (Vass, Short, Pratt.)

Dogs lose relatively more via the lungs directly (and the mucus membrane of the mouth), for they pant when they are too hot. Their skin loss is concentrated in the pads of their feet.

Clinically I find the above of little importance, at least as far as the lung-skin relationship is concerned. Patients who feel too hot or too cold, or where a part of the body is subjectively too hot or too cold, may have a hyper or hypoactivity of any of the twelve basic organs; other symptoms and signs are normally a better guide.

The thermoregulatory function of the kidney should not be forgotten.

Symptomatology

Main Meridian Symptoms

The chest is distended, dyspnoea, coughing, pain in the supra-clavicular fossa going down to the thumb or index finger. When severe, blurred vision, palms of hands hot, palpitations, polydipsia.

SYMPTOMS OF EXCESS

Upper part of the back and shoulder ache, the patient feels superficially cold, perspiration and fainting, micturition frequent but in small amounts.

SYMPTOMS OF INSUFFICIENCY

Upper part of back and shoulders painful and cold, gasping for breath, colour of urine changes.

Lung Cold Symptoms

If the lungs are invaded by cold evil, this may cause the lungs to lose the function of Qi transformation, with the result that fluids are not transformed and digested.

This causes coughing, dyspnoea, excessive phlegm, lack of thirst. Possibly the chest is distended, with constant coughing, inability to lie down, and oedema of the whole body including the face and round the eyes.

The pulse is floating and wiry, possibly wiry and slippery.

The tongue is white and slippery.

Lung Hot Symptoms

May be caused by dry evil or dry heat, or cold which has become extreme and therefore has changed to fire, producing heat symptoms.

The symptoms of lung heat are fever with a red face, both cheeks red, mental agitation, thirsty even after drinking, throat red and painful, stools dry hard and dense, urine dark, nose slightly red, epistaxis, coughing and vomiting of thick mucous, possibly the mucous is streaked with blood, pain in chest and back during coughing, throat feels blocked and constricted, possibly tonsillitis.

The pulse is slippery and rapid.
The tongue is dry and yellow.

Lung Empty Symptoms

The condition lung empty may entail either lung Qi empty or lung Yin empty.

The main symptoms of lung Qi empty are:—breathing light, voice weak, sweating, throat and head dry, face shiny and white, skin dry, hair on head comes out easily, frequent micturition, body fears the cold, easily catches colds, influenza, pneumonia, etc. In addition there may be long periods of coughing and dyspnoea, difficult breathing and the patient may lack strength.

The pulse is empty and fine, the right inch pulse being particularly weak.

The tongue substance is pale red.

The principal symptoms of lung Yin empty are:—flushing and spontaneous sweating, both cheeks red, throat dry and mouth parched, violent coughing, slow and heavy coughing. In some cases the throat may be painful and the voice very weak; there may be haemoptysis, and the body may become increasingly emaciated.

The pulse is empty, fine and rapid, or hollow and rapid.

The tongue substance is deep red.

Lung Full Symptoms

If wind cold full evil blocks and restricts the lungs, then the lung Qi is obstructed and does not penetrate, causing dyspnoea and distension of the chest. The pulse is slippery and full.

If lung Qi is abundant, then there is coughing and Qi rises, the shoulders and back are painful, and there is sweating.

If fluid is stopped, then there is dry coughing and shortness of breath, pain in chest whilst coughing.

If phlegm is hot, then there will be continuous coughing and Qi rises. In severe cases, there is purulent phlegm with a foul smell, and distension of the chest. The pulse is rapid and full.

Connecting Meridian (Luo) Symptoms

SYMPTOMS OF EXCESS

Lower end of radius and palm of hands both hot.

Coughing, yawning with mouth wide open, constant desire to urinate.

Muscle Meridian Symptoms

Muscular spasm, pain and dysfunction along the course of the meridian. Haemoptysis with pains in the sides.

Course of Meridians

Lung Main Meridian

Principal Course

From L1 below the clavicle, the meridian arches over the front of the shoulder, to descend along the embryologically anterior and outer surface of the arm, terminating at the end of the thumb at L11.

Special Details

The meridian starts in the middle warmer stomach area, deep to Cv12. It descends to loop around the transverse colon, with which it is connected at the level of Cv9; ascends again to Cv13, passing the pylorus and the cardia of the stomach. It penetrates the diaphragm and enters the lungs to which it belongs (?represented by Cv17), rising to the level of the larynx. Here it passes horizontally to emerge at L1, and thence goes down the arm to L11.

A branch goes from L7 along the outer side of the index finger to L11.

Lung Connecting Meridian (Luo)—L7

This meridian follows the course of the main meridian and enters the palm of the hand. From L7 it diverges to connect with the Luo of the large intestine.

Lung Muscle Meridian

The meridian begins at the end of the thumb, unites at the wrist; ascends the forearm, unites at the elbow; ascends the upper arm, enters the chest, emerging at the sterno-clavicular joint where it unites; goes across the clavicle to unite at the front of the shoulder. It descends and unites inside the chest, and is dispersed as far as the diaphragm.

Important Points

Wood	L11	
Fire	L10	
Earth	L9	Tonification
Metal	L8	Metal point of Yin metal meridian
Water	L5	Sedation
Source	L9	
Luo	L7	
Xi	L6	
Alarm	L1	
Associated	B13	

CHAPTER III

LARGE INTESTINE

Traditional Chinese and Western Scientific Conceptions

'The Large Intestine Controls the Transmitting and Drainage of the Dregs'

According to Chinese conceptions:

The stomach controls the receiving, rotting and ripening (digestion) of liquid and solid food.

The spleen controls the moving, transforming and distribution of the pure essence of the already rotted and ripened liquid and solid food, to all parts of the body, in order to nourish it.

The small intestine takes the waste materials of the liquid digestate and via the bladder expels them through the urethra.

The large intestine takes the remaining solid dregs and expels them via the anus. The large intestine takes the surplus of the solid matter and expels it at the appropriate time, having the functions of: transmission, drainage of dregs and control of defaecation.

Thus the small intestine has the function of dividing the food and water into the 'pure and impure', *i.e.*, the relationship of micturition defaecation. It can quite often be observed that patients who have diarrhoea pass little urine, while those who are constipated pass more urine. It follows from this that one type of diarrhoea may be treated either by stimulating the large intestine or by increasing the flow of urine.

The Lung and Large Intestine

The lung and large intestine have coupled meridians and thus influence one another. In pneumonia there is usually constipation, though occasionally diarrhoea. Conversely, with constipation there is often dyspnoea with distension of the chest, which is cured when the constipation is cured. That the lung and large intestine are coupled organs, or as the Chinese say, have an interior-exterior relationship, both under the jurisdiction of the element metal, may seem a little peculiar to the Westerner. The astute observer will notice clinical correlations, such as those mentioned in the above sentences. The following examples from embryology and comparative anatomy shed some light on the problem.

The large intestine and lungs are both derived from entoderm: The large intestine is formed from the caudal part of the primitive gut; the lung bud, which develops into the bronchial system, is a ventral evagination of the primitive foregut.

In fish the inner portion of the gill clefts (pulmonary function) is also formed from the primitive gut—albeit the opposite end to the colon.

In many larvae and embryos of fish, before the definitive gills have developed as an organ for the assimilation of oxygen from the water, this function is performed by the blood vessels in the yolk sac (which is the external part of the primitive gut) and the fin folds (fin folds are skin, which comes under the metal organs). The more favourable the respiratory conditions under which the embryos and larvae develop, the less strongly developed is their capillary respiratory system. As the yolk sac is absorbed and its respiratory blood vessel network is reduced, there is a corresponding increase in the blood vessel network in the fin folds. (Nikolsky and Soin, 1954.) This fin fold respiration is part of the lung/large intestine, skin and respiration complex, partly discussed in the section on the lungs.

There is intestinal respiration among Cuprinoids (sheat-fish, loaches) and Symbranchidae. In these the length of the intestine is increased with the capillary network nearer the internal mucosal surface. In some parts of the gut there is complete absence of digestive function and intestinal villi.

In the tropical sheat-fish, Otocinchus, there is a special blind outgrowth from the stomach, usually full of air, which performs a respiratory function.

Swallowed air in the fish loses about 5% of its oxygen and acquires about 3% of carbon dioxide. Human pulmonary respiration is more effective as about 25% of the inspired oxygen is absorbed and the exhaled air contains about 4% carbon dioxide (dry air at sea level contains 0.04 volumes per cent). The used air in the fish leaves, either through the mouth as in many sheat-fish, or through the anus as in the loach.

The Nose, Throat and Teeth

The nose, throat and the teeth are to some extent controlled by the large intestine, particularly those regions covered by the meridian.

Case History. A patient had a clear nasal discharge. This was cured by stimulating the large intestine at Li4. In other patients Li20 gives a better result.

Haemorrhage

According to Soulié de Morant, there is an increased tendency to bleed when the large intestine is under-active. This could possibly be explained by the biosynthesis of vitamin K in the colon. Supposedly menorrhagia can for this reason be treated by stimulating the large intestine.

In my experience pernicious anaemia cannot be treated via the large intestine, despite the fact that vitamin B12 is made there by bacterial action.

Symptomatology

Main Meridian Symptoms

Toothache, swelling of the neck, diseases associated with Fluid which this meridian controls, discolouration of the eyes, dry mouth, clear flow of mucus from the nose, epistaxis, sore throat, pain in shoulder arm thumb and forefinger.

SYMPTOMS OF EXCESS

Warmth or swelling along the course of the meridian.

SYMPTOMS OF INSUFFICIENCY

Cold, shivering with difficulty in getting warm again.

Large Intestine Cold Symptoms

If the large intestine is cold then the waste products that it expels will be cold, with relatively little smell. Abdomen painful with borborygmi, urine clear, diarrhoea, hands and feet cold.

The pulse is deep and slow.

The tongue fur is white and slippery.

Large Intestine Hot Symptoms

If the large intestine is hot, then the mouth is dry and the lips are scorched, with constipation, rectal pain and a feeling of swelling. If there is damp heat, then the stools are often loose and foul smelling. If the condition is severe, they are reddish-brown, and dark urine is passed in small quantities. If the disease persists for a long time, it may result in Zang intoxication. If the blood is hot and the blood vessels are injured, there will be blood in the stools.

The pulse is rapid.

The tongue fur is yellow and dry.

Large Intestine Empty Symptoms

If the large intestine Qi is empty, there is prolapse of the rectum. This occurs more easily in women if they exert too much pressure during labour, or it may occur if the Qi is weak after prolonged dysentery. In each case the limbs are cold.

The pulse is fine and minute.

Large Intestine Full Symptoms

If the stomach is full and hot, and this moves into the large intestine, then there will be constipation, painful abdomen, thirst, incoherent speech.

The pulse is deep and full.

The tongue fur is dry, yellow and greasy.

If damp poison and heat combine in the large intestine, then the lower abdomen is painful, which is worse when pressed, stools moist and bloody, alternately cold and hot, with sweating.

The pulse is slippery and rapid.

If summer heat and damp evils combine and form a blockage together with food and drink in the large intestine and this becomes dysentery, then the abdomen is painful, with a great desire to defaecate.

Connecting Meridian (Luo) Symptoms

SYMPTOMS OF EXCESS

Dental caries, deafness.

SYMPTOMS OF INSUFFICIENCY

Teeth cold, diaphragmatic area feels as if it is blocked.

Muscle Meridian Symptoms

Muscular spasm, pain and dysfunction along the course of the meridian muscle. Cannot raise shoulders, cannot turn head.

Course of Meridians

Large Intestine Main Meridian

Principal Course

The meridian starts on the index finger at Li1. It goes up the embryologically posterior and outer surface of the arm, over the shoulder neck and jaw, to end at the side of the nose at Li20.

Special Details

From Li14 to T13.

From Li16 the meridian goes (? via Si12) to Gv14 and thence over the shoulder to S12. From here it passes through the lungs, with which it is connected, penetrates the diaphragm and enters the large intestine, to which it belongs, at S25.

The branch meridian leaves S12 to go to Li17, Li18 (? via S7), Gv26 and then across the midline to Li19 and Li20 on the opposite side.

From the region of S7 through the lower jaws and teeth to the region of Cv24.

(? From Li20 to S4 and G14.)

Large Intestine Connecting Meridian (Luo)—Li6

The meridian begins above the wrist at Li6, runs along the arm, goes over the shoulder and jaw and connects with the teeth and ears. It combines with the ?Zong Mo in this region. It links with the lung meridian Luo.

Large Intestine Muscle Meridian

The meridian begins at the end of the index finger, unites at the wrist; ascends the arm, unites at the elbow; ascends the upper arm, unites at the shoulder. A branch goes over the shoulder blade then going up and down the spine. The main muscle meridian ascends over the shoulder and neck in front of the small intestine muscle meridian, then up the lateral side of the forehead and temple, over the summit of the head, to descend on the opposite side as far as the jaw. A branch from the neck ascends the jaw, to unite at the side of the nose.

Large Intestine and Lung Divergent Meridians

Large Intestine Divergent Meridian

The large intestine divergent meridian leaves the large intestine main meridian at the outer tip of the shoulder. It goes to the spinal column and thence over the shoulder, thorax and upper abdomen to the large intestine to which it belongs and also to the lungs. It emerges at the supra-clavicular fossa, going along the throat to the large intestine meridian.

Lung Divergent Meridian

The lung divergent meridian leaves the lung main meridian at the armpit, whence it enters the lungs and scatters in the large intestine. Above this, it emerges from the supra-clavicular fossa, follows the throat and again meets the large intestine meridian.

Important Points

Metal	Li1	Metal point of Yang metal meridian
Water	Li2	Sedation
Wood	Li3	
Fire	Li5	
Earth	Li11	Tonification
Source	Li4	
Luo	Li6	
Xi	Li7	
Alarm	S25	
Associated	B25	

CHAPTER IV

STOMACH

Traditional Chinese and Western Scientific Conceptions

The Digestive Function of the Stomach

The Stomach is called 'the sea of water and nourishment and the controller of the rotting and ripening of liquid and solid food'.

The Jing Qi which is required to nourish the organs of the body is produced by the 'rotting and ripening' of food and liquid in the stomach. Without the nourishing action of the Jing Qi, the other organs of the body could not function.

'*The stomach is the sea of the five Zang and six Fu; liquid and solid food enter the stomach and the five Zang and six Fu are endowed with Qi from the stomach.*'

(Ling Shu, wuwei pian)

The Jing Qi produced in the stomach and distributed to the other organs is stored in the kidney. This stored Jing can be used to nourish the organs and can also be transformed to the Jing of sexual power and semen. It is therefore said:

'*The kidneys are the root of the former heaven (pre-natal). The spleen and stomach are the root of latter heaven (post-natal).*'

The kidney semen-Jing gives the stimulus to birth. The stomach-Jing is required for growth.

The digestive function of gastric juice, particularly pepsinogen, is well known. The stomach may even digest itself in a healthy person who dies suddenly after a meal.

The Stomach and Spleen

The stomach and spleen are coupled organs, and as such their function is mutually interdependent. While the stomach controls the rotting and ripening of food and water, the spleen controls the 'moving and transforming' of food and water, and transports and distributes Jing Qi and fluid.

The spleen is a Yin Zang, the stomach is a Yang Fu. The spleen is damp earth, dislikes damp and likes dryness. The stomach is dry earth, dislikes dryness and likes moisture. For the spleen, the ascent of Qi is normal; for the stomach, the descent of Qi is normal.

If the spleen does not move and transform, then the stomach cannot digest; if the stomach does not rot and ripen water and food, the spleen cannot move and transform. If the spleen is empty and accumulates damp, then this can distress and check stomach Yang, and can produce a distended abdomen with anorexia. If the stomach is dry and hot, this will dry up the spleen's fluid, and can produce the symptoms of dry mouth and lips, owing to the spleen's fluid not having the means of ascending and moistening the mouth.

Vomiting may be caused by a malfuntion of stomach Qi which has lost its normal function of descending, and instead rebels upwards. In diarrhoea, the spleen has lost its strength and movement and power to ascend, thereby allowing descent and diarrhoea.

The stomach is influenced by abnormal hunger or satiation, or by an excess of cold or hot foods.

From the point of view of Western medicine there is no association in function between the stomach and spleen. They are though in intimate contact, not only in man but also in most fishes, amphibians, birds and mammals. In the dogfish the spleen is attached by a membrane to the hinder end of the stomach as a triangular lobe with a forward prolongation along the right side of the pyloric division. In the pigeon the spleen is attached to the right side of the proventriculus. In the rabbit the spleen is a narrow, crescentic body lying on the convex side of the stomach.

The Salivary Glands

The salivary glands are influenced by stimulation of the stomach meridian, which passes over the parotid gland between S2 and S3, and over the submaxillary gland between S8 and S9.

Saliva assists the stomach, by the digestion of starches with ptyalin, by the lubrication of food, and by making it possible to taste food, which is only possible if the tongue is moist.

In poisonous snakes the action of saliva goes beyond digestion to that of killing its prospective meal, for the poison glands are modified parotid glands.

The Tongue

The tongue is used as an important diagnostic criterion in Chinese

Traditional Medicine, whole books being entirely devoted to this subject.

The fur on the tongue principally reflects the condition of the stomach or, indirectly, the effect of other organs such as the liver on the stomach.

The mucous membrane covering the tongue is derived from entoderm, just as the lining of the whole of the gastro-intestinal tract. The oral membrane divides the tongue of the embryo into an internal and external portion in front of the row of vallate papillae, the former being covered by entoderm, the latter by ectoderm. At a later stage of embryonic development though, the entoderm covering the root of the tongue slips forward to coat the whole of the body as well.

Case History. A patient was seen whose tongue was covered with a white greasy fur. She was able to eat only small amounts of food at a time and had frequent epigastric pain or discomfort.

Pulse diagnosis showed a dysfunction of the stomach and this was cured by treating S36.

Symptomatology

Main Meridian Symptoms

Shivering with cold, constant yawning, dark complexion. When the disease is serious, the patient hates other people, is alarmed when hearing the sound of leaves rustling, has palpitations, and wishes to close the doors and windows and live by himself in the house. In severe cases, he may ascend to high places and sing, take off his clothes and run away. Abdomen distended, intermittent fevers, warm diseases, Shen confused, leading to madness, followed by fever. Spontaneous sweating, clear nasal discharge, epistaxis, mouth awry, mouth and lips develop dry sores, swelling of neck, ascites, pain or disturbance of function along the course of the meridian, especially the second and third toe.

SYMPTOMS OF EXCESS

Front of body hot. The heat in the stomach dissolves the liquid and solid food causing hunger and thirst. Yellow urine.

SYMPTOMS OF INSUFFICIENCY

The front of the body is cold and shivering. When the stomach is cold, the abdomen will be swollen and full.

Stomach Cold Symptoms

If the stomach Yang is deficient and cold Qi is dominant, this may cause the stomach to become distended and painful, the pain being continuous, with heartburn and waterbrash. When more severe, there will be vomiting and hiccoughs. Possibly there is very severe pain, with a desire for heat and pressure on the stomach. Possibly the limbs are cold.

The pulse of the right 2nd position is deep and slow.

The tongue has white and slippery fur.

Stomach Hot Symptoms

If the stomach fire is excessive, then the fluid in the stomach is easily destroyed, giving rise to a parched mouth, polydipsia, a feeling of hunger and discomfort, foul smell from mouth, bleeding from gums, gingivitis, vomiting immediately after meals. If the stomach heat moves down into the large intestine, then defaecation is often difficult, and if severe the stools become dry, and there is constipation.

Stomach Empty Symptoms

If the stomach Qi is empty, then the upper abdomen and lower chest feel blocked and melancholic or painful; there is no desire to eat and possibly belching; food is not digested, and there may be diarrhoea. If the condition is severe, then undigested food is passed and lips and tongue become pale white. If the fluid in the stomach is deficient, this can produce chocking or inability to swallow food.

The pulse in the 2nd position right is weak and pliable.

Stomach Full Symptoms

Stomach full symptoms are usually produced in externally contracted diseases and are Fu full symptoms. As the stomach and intestines are full and hot, there is pain in the abdomen and constipation; if the food is not digested, then there is abdominal distension and pain, sour and putrid vomitus, constipation, or possibly mild diarrhoea.

The pulse is full and large.

The tongue is thickly covered with yellow fur.

Connecting Meridian (Luo) Symptoms

SYMPTOMS OF EXCESS

Sudden loss of speech, insanity.

SYMPTOMS OF INSUFFICIENCY

Feet flaccid and weak, flesh and skin on shins withered and shrunken.

Muscle Meridian Symptoms

Spasm of the middle three toes and along the tibia, front of thigh swollen, herniae, muscular spasm of abdominal muscles or of the jaw, facial paralysis. If the muscles affecting the jaw are cold, there is muscular spasm extending from the jaw to the mouth. If they are hot, then the muscles are flaccid and cannot contract, therefore the mouth droops. According to circumstances it may be impossible to open or close the eyes.

Course of Meridians

Stomach Main Meridian

Principal Course

The meridian starts at S1, going over the face and the forehead, over the chest, and along the embryologically posterior and outer surface of the leg to end at the tip of the second toe at S45. According to some accounts the meridian starts at S1, going to S2, S3 (angle of jaw), S4 (below the eye), S5, S6, S7 (angle of mouth), S8 (jaw), S9 (larynx), etc. According to other accounts the meridian starts at S4 (below the eye) going to S5, S6, S7 (angle of mouth), S8, S3, S2, S1 (angle of forehead), the main meridian continuing downward to the larynx at S9 from a point slightly anterior to S8.

Special Details

The meridian starts at the side of the nose at Li20, goes to the midline just below the bridge of the nose to meet its companion from the other side, and then goes on to B1, S4, S5, S6, Gv26, S7, Cv24, S8, S3, S2, G3, G6, G5, G4, S1, (? via G14) to Gv24. From S8 to S9, S10, S11 (? over the shoulders to Gv14 and thence forward again) to S12. Thence over the chest and abdomen to S30, and down the leg to end at the lateral tip of the second toe at S45.

A branch leaves S12, descends to the diaphragm, and enters the stomach, to which it belongs, at Cv13, and connects with the spleen.

A branch leaves Cv12 at the pylorus and moves inside the abdomen down to S30.

A branch leaves S36 going lateral to the main meridian, to end at the lateral tip of the third toe.

A branch leaves S42 going to Sp1.

According to classical accounts, the whole of the main meridian below S8 is described as a branch.

Stomach Connecting Meridian (Luo)—S40

The meridian begins in the lower leg at S40, ascends to reach the head and nape of neck where it combines with the meridian Qi of all the other meridians and descends to connect with the throat. It links with the spleen meridian Luo.

Stomach Muscle Meridian

The meridian begins at the 3rd toe (possible also 2nd and 4th toe), unites at the ankle; ascends the lower leg and unites at the outer side of the knee; continues up to unit at the hip joint; crosses the ribs and joins the spinal column to which it belongs. The main muscle meridian ascends from the ankle to unite at the antero-lateral side of the knee. A branch from here goes laterally to unite with the gall-bladder muscle meridian. The main muscle meridian ascends past S32 to unite at the top of the thigh; accumulates in the genitalia; ascends and scatters in the abdomen; and unites in the supra-clavicular fossa. It ascends at the side of the neck and mouth to meet at the side of the nose and then unites at the nose. It ascends to meet the bladder muscle meridian; the bladder muscle meridian running supra-orbitally, and the stomach muscle meridian mainly infra-orbitally. A branch from the jaw unites in front of the ear.

Stomach and Spleen Divergent Meridians

Stomach Divergent Meridian

The stomach divergent meridian leaves the main stomach meridian at the middle of the thigh; thereafter it enters the abdomen and goes to the stomach to which it belongs, and thence disperses in the spleen. Thereafter it ascends further to penetrate the heart and continues along the throat to emerge at the mouth. Thence it goes round the ala of the nose to the bridge of the nose between the eyes, with which it is linked, and there it meets the main stomach meridian.

Spleen Divergent Meridian

The spleen divergent meridian leaves the spleen main meridian at the middle of the thigh, thereafter it follows the course of the stomach divergent meridian to the throat, where it penetrates the middle of the tongue.

Important Points

Metal	S45	Sedation
Water	S44	
Wood	S43	
Fire	S41	Tonification
Earth	S36	Earth point of Yang earth meridian
Source	S42	
Luo	S40	
Xi	S34	
Alarm	Cv12	
Associated	B21	

CHAPTER V

SPLEEN

Traditional Chinese and Western Scientific Conceptions

The Spleen's Function of Distributing Nourishment

The principal function of the spleen is to move and transport the Jing Qi of liquid and solid food, and to distribute the Jing Qi around the whole body.

'*Drink enters the stomach, the Jing Qi overflows, and it is transported to the spleen. The Spleen Qi scatters the Jing.*'

(Su Wen, jingmo bielun)

'*The spleen controls the movement of fluid in the stomach.*'

(Su Wen, juelun)

Jing Qi and fluid are the two essential nourishing substances and, although they are first processed in the stomach, they are further transformed and also distributed by the spleen.

'*The spleen meridian is earth, and only this Zang irrigates the four sides.*'

(Su Wen, yuji zhenzang lun)

This is the phenomenon of 'earth creates the myriad things' applied to the function of the spleen.

If the moving and transforming ability of the spleen is deficient, the refined parts of the food cannot be transported to each part of the body, and the symptoms of fullness of the abdomen, borborygmi, diarrhoea, non-digestion of food, and possibly loss of appetite will appear. There will also be the symptoms which arise from these, such as emaciation of flesh, Jing Shen weary, etc.

The spleen moves and transforms not only the fine parts of the food, but also those of liquid. If the spleen Qi is empty and weak and loses its moving and transforming ability, this can lead to disease. For example, if the water in the stomach and intestines is not absorbed, this will cause diarrhoea and oliguria. If the water in the flesh and skin does not escape, then the body will be heavy and the skin swollen.

Case History. A patient had generalised subcutaneous oedema; it was not more marked in one part of the body than another. Her abdomen felt distended, she was depressed and lethargic, she sometimes had symptoms similar to those of a deep vein thrombosis of the leg. All symptoms and signs were helped by giving diuretics. The results though were only temporary.

Pulse diagnosis showed an underactive spleen. She was considerably improved, though not completely cured, by stimulating Sp3.

The Spleen Governs the Blood

Many blood diseases are related in one way or another to the spleen, *e.g.*, continuous defaecation of blood (?), polymenorrhoea, dysmenorrhoea, etc. In these cases, one should 'lead the blood back to the spleen, and tonify the spleen so that it unites the blood'.

As is well known, there is a splenomegaly in certain anaemias. The spleen also takes part in the destruction of erythrocytes, the regulation of blood flow in the portal system, the function of a blood reservoir, the conversion of haemoglobin to ferritin and bilirubin-globin, the formation of lymphocytes and monocytes, and haematopoiesis in the embryo.

The Spleen, Flesh, and Lips

'Now if the spleen is diseased, it cannot move the fluid on behalf of the stomach. The four limbs are thus not able to obtain the Qi of liquid and solid food. Hence the Qi decays gradually. The meridian cannot function correctly and the muscles, bones, skin and flesh have no Qi with which to grow, and therefore they do not function.'

(Su Wen, taiyin yangmin lun)

The above quotation explains, via the theories of traditional Chinese medicine, why weakness or emaciation of the skin, flesh or limbs are diseases that are dependent upon the spleen.

Likewise, the redness and the moisture of the lips and mouth is also dependent upon the spleen. Patients who have a weak digestion due to an under-activity of the spleen usually have pale red and dry lips, and the mucous membrane lining of their mouth has a greyish tinge.

Yin earth likes dryness and hates damp. If the spleen is empty, water and dampness are not transformed. If there is an abundance of dampness, the spleen earth will suffer, producing amongst other symptoms large loose stools that float on water.

The Spleen and Pancreas

From the above, mainly translations of Chinese texts, it is obvious that many of the functions ascribed to the spleen really belong to the pancreas. For this reason many French doctors call this the Spleen-Pancreas meridian.

The external secretions of the pancreas—trypsin, chymotrypsin, carboxypeptidase, amylase, maltase, lipase—account for many of the previously mentioned symptoms. The internal secretion of the pancreas—insulin—may probably account for the other symptoms, such as wasting of the flesh.

Anatomically the spleen and pancreas are closer together than one might think, for both are developed in the dorsal mesogastrium, a connection that is virtually lost in the adult. Accessory spleens or pancreases occur in much the same region.

I do not know of any digestive function of the spleen, or even one concerning the distribution of the products of digestion, though this may one day be found. At least the spleen is distended after a meal and it belongs to the portal circulation, as do other organs associated with digestion.

Obsession and Concentration

The spleen seems occasionally to be connected with obsessions. The person who goes back twice to see if he has locked his front door, or who always insists on doing something in a certain way, may have a splenic dysfunction.

Excessive sympathy or over-concentration may be associated with the spleen or the stomach, as seen in one type of duodenal ulcer.

Symptomatology

Main Meridian Symptoms

Root of tongue stiff and hard, vomiting on eating, epigastrium tender, abdomen distended, continuous belching, difficulty in swallowing food, feels great relief and contentment on defaecating or breaking wind, dysentery, stools thin and watery, ascites, jaundice, body aching and heavy, cannot lie down peacefully, inner side of knees and thighs become swollen and cold if forced to stand for a long time, difficulty in moving big toe, palpitations, cardiac pain, cold intermittent fevers, feeling of oppression in chest, sharp pain below the heart, abdomen distended due to constipation, oliguria.

SYMPTOMS OF EXCESS

Pain in abdomen.

SYMPTOMS OF INSUFFICIENCY

Abdomen distended and taut like a drum.

Spleen Cold Symptoms

If the spleen Yang is deficient and cannot move and transform water and damp, thus causing Yin cold to become dominant, then clinically one may see continuous pain in the abdomen, clear cold diarrhoea, inability to digest food and drink, cold limbs, heavy body. The skin may be yellow-black, the whole body may be swollen and puffy; oliguria may be present.

The pulse is deep and slow, particularly the right 2nd position.

The tongue is furred white and is greasy.

Spleen Hot Symptoms

The spleen is basically damp earth; if heat is associated with it, then damp and heat contend with each other, and the face becomes swollen and red and bloated. The body is heavy, there is a feeling of melancholy in the chest, and some anorexia, it is relatively easy to become jaundiced, urine is dark and in small amounts; there may be hot dysentery with abdominal pain that is not constant, lips may be red, and the mouth may have a sweet sticky and dirty taste.

Spleen Empty Symptoms

If spleen earth is empty and weak, and its transporting function is impaired, there will be a concomitant decrease in the desire to eat and drink, or there will be difficulty in digestion after eating. There is vomiting with a swollen abdomen, borborygmi and loose stools, four limbs cold, weariness and fondness for lying down, abdomen painful with a desire to press it, possibly emaciation and at the same time oedema.

The pulse is empty and slowed down, specially so in the right connecting position.

The tongue substance is pale, with white and slippery fur.

Spleen Full Symptoms

If the spleen is full, then there are usually diseases caused by damp evil remaining, and the symptoms are opposite to those of spleen empty symptoms.

If damp obstructs and blocks communication, then the upper abdomen is full and distended; if damp remains in the skin and flesh, then the body will feel heavy; if damp obstructs Qi, there will be oligura and constipation, weak respiration, with a melancholic feeling in the chest, and a feeling of fullness, pain, and possibly swelling in the abdomen.

Connecting Meridian (Luo) Symptoms

SYMPTOMS OF EXCESS
Sharp pain in intestines.

SYMPTOMS OF INSUFFICIENCY
Ascites.

Great Luo of the Spleen—Sp21—Symptoms

SYMPTOMS OF EXCESS
Whole body painful.

SYMPTOMS OF INSUFFICIENCY
Bones and joints of the whole body flaccid and weak and without strength.

Muscle Meridian Symptoms

Pain or muscular spasm in big toe, inner side of knee, inner side of thigh, genitalia, navel and ribs.   Pain along the spine extending to the breast.

Course of Meridians

Spleen Main Meridian

Principal Course

Starting at Sp1 on the big toe, the meridian goes up the embryological anterior and outer surface of the leg, over the abdomen and chest to the axilla at Sp20, and then down a little to Sp21.

Special Details

The meridian starts at Sp1 and goes up the leg to the groin at Sp13.
From Sp13 via Cv3 and Cv4 to Sp14.
From Sp15 via Cv10 to Sp16.

From Sp16 via G24 and Liv14 to Sp17, and thence on to Sp21.

From Sp21 via L1, up the throat to end on the under surface of the tongue.

A branch leaves Cv10, penetrates the diaphragm and goes to the heart and heart meridian.

Traditionally, from Sp13 the meridian is described as entering the abdomen, going to the spleen to which it belongs, and connecting with the stomach.

Spleen Connecting Meridian (Luo)—Sp4

The meridian begins near the root of the big toe at Sp4 and ascends to enter the abdomen, connecting with the intestines and stomach. It links with the stomach meridian Luo.

Great Luo of the Spleen—Sp21

The meridian begins on the side of the chest below the axilla at Sp21, and then divides and disperses throughout the chest and ribs.

This connecting meridian unites all the Yin and Yang Luo like a net and if there is any 'extravasated blood' it should be treated at Sp21.

Spleen Muscle Meridian

The meridian begins on the medial side of the end of the big toe, unites at the internal malleolus; ascends to unite at the medial side of the knee; ascends the medial surface of the thigh to unite at its upper end; accumulates in the genitalia; ascends the abdomen to unite at the navel; crosses the abdomen to unite at the ribs, and scatters in the chest. An inner branch ascends the spine.

Important Points

Wood	Sp1	
Fire	Sp2	Tonification
Earth	Sp3	Earth point of Yin earth meridian
Metal	Sp5	Sedation
Water	Sp9	
Source	Sp3	
Luo	Sp4	
Xi	Sp8	
Alarm	Liv13	
Associated	B20	

CHAPTER VI

HEART

Traditional Chinese and Western Scientific Conceptions

'The Heart is the Ruling Organ and Controller of the Shen Ming'

The heart is the controller of life and movement in the body, and occupies the first place among the Zang and Fu. All Jing Shen, consciousness and thought are connected with the function of the heart; it is called therefore the 'ruling official (or organ)'.

'The heart is the supreme controller of the five Zang and the six Fu, and is the dwelling place of the Jing Shen.'

(Ling Shu, xieke pian)

'The heart is the root of life, and the location of change of Shen.'

(Su Wen, liujie zangziang lun)

These quotations explain that the heart includes the function of Shen, leads the movement of the Zang and Fu, and is the controller of life and movement; the ancients thus stressed the importance of the function of the heart. Clinical experience shows that, if the heart becomes diseased, one may have the symptoms of palpitations, nervousness, insomnia, delirium, incoherent speech, confused Shen Zhi, liability to sorrow, incessant laughter, etc. The causes of these conditions have two aspects; inner injury and outer suffering. Inner injury is present if the heart itself is not strong, or when excessive emotions (happiness, melancholy, fear, worry) cause disease. Outer suffering is present if the 'six excess disease evils' invade, if evil heat rebels and is transmitted to the pericardium, etc. However, the principal cause is still that the heart's action has lost its control.

Since the heart is 'the great controller' of the Zang and Fu, it can 'unite and lead the division of work, and the working together of the Zang and Fu; moreover it can reciprocally obtain harmony and produce the functional co-ordination of the whole body.' If each organ honours its office, the health of the body will be maintained. Conversely, if the heart is diseased, then the movement of the other Zang and Fu will be in disorder, and thus the health of the whole body is affected, and at all times there is the possibility of disease.

'*Thus if the controller is bright, there is peace . . . if the controller is not bright, then the twelve organs are in danger.*'

(Su Wen, linglan midian lun)

Case History. A patient had variable symptoms one day in one part of the body, another day in another part.

Pulse diagnosis showed a different disturbance every time the pulse was felt. The overall quality of the pulse was always the same; the specific abnormalities shifting from one pulse position to another. The pulse position of the heart did not show any greater abnormality than any other position. This variable symptomatology nevertheless suggested the heart as the main culprit, and when this was treated the condition was largely cured.

The Heart Controls the Blood Vessels, its Exterior Reflexion is in the Face

The blood vessels are one of the 'five substances', and their function is to enclose the blood and cause it to circulate constantly round the whole body. This circulation, though, is controlled by the heart.

'*The heart is the root of life . . . its exterior reflection is in the face, its interior reflection is in the blood vessels.*'

(Su Wen, zangziang lun)

If the heart and blood vessels are 'bloodless', the face has a grey ashen colour.

'*If the arm lesser Yin (heart) Qi is interrupted, then the blood vessels will not function; if the vessels do not function, then the blood does not flow; if the blood does not flow, then the hair and skin are not moistened. Thus the face will be black like lacquer wood and the blood will die.*'

(Ling Shu, jingmo pian)

The phylogenetic and ontogenetic development of the heart as a specialisation of the blood vessels need hardly be mentioned. In fish the heart is little more than the hypertrophied muscular wall of the aorta. In the human embryo primitive blood vessels appear first— and these are only later modified to form a heart.

Case History. A patient of 28 had mitral incompetence. The heart was enlarged; the apex beat could easily be seen, let alone felt; he could only walk a few hundred yards and then stopped because of tingling in his hands and dyspnoea. He perspired profusely.

Pulse diagnosis showed an abnormality not only of the heart but also of the liver and kidney. After eight treatments the patient went without my knowledge on the C.N.D. Aldermaston march to London (30 miles). He did this with no more difficulty than any of the other marchers of his age.

Presumably the effect of acupuncture was to increase the function of the heart so that it was able to compensate for the mitral incompetence. It should be stressed that such a good result, in an irreparable structural lesion, can only be obtained in a small proportion of patients.

The Relationship Between the Heart and the Tongue

A red or a deep red tongue generally indicates that the heart is hot, and that fire Qi has a surplus. A pale red tongue shows that blood is empty, and that the heart Qi is deficient. If the Shen of the heart receives disease, this can cause a feeble tongue and inability to speak.

'(*Heart*) *its influence reaches to the tongue.*'

(Su Wen, yinyang yingxiang dalun)

'*The heart Qi communicates with the tongue; if the heart is harmonious, then the tongue is able to recognise the five tastes.*'

(Ling Shu, modu pian)

The tongue and heart are much nearer to one another in the embryo than in the adult, the heart being more or less in the neck.

In the embryo the heart is connected with the region of the base of the tongue by the dorsal mesocardium, a proximity which is probably not fortuitous.

Case History. A patient was seen whose leading symptom was tingling at the tip of the tongue, which had been constant and unremittant for many years. On close questioning she had slight retrosternal discomfort and dyspnoea on extention.

Pulse diagnosis showed an underactivity of the heart. She was cured by stimulating various points on the heart meridian.

The Thyroid and Heart

In Chinese pulse diagnosis, hyperthyroidism is shown by the pulse of the heart (position 1, deep, left) becoming distended and hard. The all too frequent over-dosage of thyroxin which physicians give their patients, in an attempt to 'pep them up', may in this way be diagnosed. The sinus tachycardia, systolic murmur, vasodilation, raised pulse pressure and paroxysmal fibrillation, which are the well-known Western cardiovasular symptoms of thyrotoxicosis, only occur at a much later stage than that noted by the more sensitive Chinese pulse diagnosis.

The endocrine glands were not known to the ancient Chinese and were therefore not considered. In view of the above though, I think the thyroid should be classified as belonging to the heart in the system of classification under twelve organs. (Likewise, as mentioned further on, the adrenal belongs to the kidney.)

Embryologically the thyroid is connected with the tongue, via the thyroglossal duct, whose remnant may be seen as the foramen caecum at the junction of the base and body of the tongue. As mentioned in the previous section the tongue is likewise connected with the heart: physiologically in the adult, anatomically in the embryo. Sometimes even the thyroid, or more frequently, aberrant parts of the thyroid, migrate downwards to lie over the pericardium.

Mild thyrotoxicos may thus be treated acupuncturally via the heart.

The Menopause

The majority of symptoms accompanying the menopause are dependent on the heart, even though Western science attaches prime importance to the ovarian hormones. Possibly one day a cardiac ovarian hormone will be discovered.

The menopause is heralded by the cessation of menstruation. Blood, which in the menopause is retained, is in the Chinese view most often classified with the heart.

The most frequent symptom of the menopause is hot flushes. Heat is traditionally classified under the heart. Palpitations and other nervous symptoms of a cardiac type may also be noted.

Patients with menopausal symptoms normally have an underactive pulse of the heart and possibly lung.

Case History. A patient was seen with severe hot flushes of several years' duration.

Pulse diagnosis showed an underactive heart and lung. She was cured in four treatments, using H7 and L9.

General

As the heart 'stores Shen' and 'controls blood', therefore it is also affected by Shen Zhi and blood. This is associated with symptoms such as palpitations, nervousness, confused Shen, delirium, haemoptysis, epistaxis, spontaneous sweating, night sweats.

Case History. A patient had pain in the region of the 5th thoracic vertebra for twenty years. Most doctors he had previously consulted thought it was a vertebral lesion, for slight arthritic changes could be seen on X-ray. On closer questioning the patient said that he felt dead elbow the level of the fifth thoracic vertebra—including his genitalia. Certainly the lower part of his body was pale while his face was bright red. There was a funnel-shaped depression over the lower part of the sternum, which was also the area where he perspired more easily than anywhere else.

Pulse diagnosis showed an overflowing heart. Treatment included H7, H5, H3, B15, B39, Gv11—all heart points. The patient was nearly, though not completely, cured.

Symptomatology

Main Meridian Symptoms

Throat dry, mouth parched, desire to drink, cardiac pain, pain in chest, pain stiffness or insensitivity down the arm along the course of the meridian, eyes yellow, palms of hands hot.

SYMPTOMS OF EXCESS

Dreams of fright, fear and anxiety.

SYMPTOMS OF INSUFFICIENCY

Inability to speak, dreams of smoke and fire.

Heart Hot Symptoms

Face red, tongue dry, tip of tongue red, pulse rapid, mouth parched, thirsty, eyes painful, under surface of tongue swollen and protruding (heavy tongue), possibly tongue swollen and hard (wooden tongue), haemoptysis, epistaxis, heart agitated and feels hot, insomnia, delirious speech, laughs incessantly, chest feels hot and melancholic, pain like a needle stab. If the heart heat moves into the small intestine, the urine becomes dark, possibly even haematuria.

Heart Empty Symptoms

Pulse generally fine and weak, tongue pale red, poor memory, nervous and not at ease often resulting in insomnia, much dreaming, dreaming that one is falling down, palpitations not only during physical exertion but even with mental effort, hurried breathing, heart seems 'noisy and hungry', violent pain below heart, pain round the lower border of the chest front and back, face withered and pale, root of tongue stiff, often sad and miserable.

A person whose heart is excessively empty is prone to sudden loss of consciousness. Other symptoms such as sweating and spermatorrhoea are also produced by the heart being empty. However, spontaneous sweating and nocturnal sweating are divided into Yin empty and Yang empty, and loss of sperm is frequently related to the kidneys, the cause being known as 'heart and kidney deficient'.

Connecting Meridian (Luo) Symptoms

SYMPTOMS OF EXCESS
Chest and diaphragmatic area feel as though they are bearing a heavy weight and are uncomfortable.

SYMPTOMS OF INSUFFICIENCY
Inability to speak.

Muscle Meridian Symptoms
Muscular spasm, pain and dysfunction along the course of the meridian. Haemoptysis.

Course of Meridians

Heart Main Meridian

Principal Course
The meridian starts in the axilla at H1, and passes along the anterior and inner surface of the arm, to end near the nail of the little finger at H9.

Special Details
The meridian emerges from the heart, to which it belongs, connects with the great vessels entering and leaving the heart, penetrates the diaphragm, and connects with the small intestine.

The main meridian leaves the heart, transversing the lung, to emerge at the armpit at H1, from where it goes down the arm to H9.

A branch from the heart goes up through the throat to the eye and contents of the orbit.

Heart Connecting Meridian (Luo)—H5

The meridian begins at H5 above the wrist, ascends alongside its main meridian and enters the heart, ascending again to link up with the root of the tongue and further to connect with the eye. It diverges and connects with the Luo of the small intestine.

Heart Muscle Meridian

The meridian begins on the little finger, unites at the wrist; ascends the forearm, unites at the elbow; ascends the upper arm, crosses the axilla where it joins the lung muscle meridian and across the anterior surface of the thorax, to unite in the middle of the chest; it runs downwards to link with the navel.

Important Points

Wood	H9	Tonification
Fire	H8	Fire point of Yin Sovereign fire meridian
Earth	H7	Sedation
Metal	H4	
Water	H3	
Source	H7	
Luo	H5	
Xi	H6	
Alarm	Cv14	
Associated	B15	

CHAPTER VII

SMALL INTESTINE

Traditional Chinese and Western Scientific Conceptions

The Small Intestine Controls the Transformation of Matter and the Separating of the Pure and Impure

'*The small intestine is the official who receives abundance and is concerned with the transforming of matter.*'

(Su Wen, linglan midian lun)

This explains that the function of the small intestine is to 'receive the water and food already rotted and ripened and sent down from the stomach, and to advance the work of separating it into the pure and impure'. It causes the Jing Qi to return to the spleen and to be distributed to the five Zang so that it may be stored there. It also causes the fluid in the 'dregs' to return to the bladder, and the solid matter to go to the large intestine, thence to be expelled from the body, thus completing the function of 'transforming matter'. Accordingly, if the function of the small intestine is not strong, it can influence micturition and defaecation.

'*Small intestine disease causes water and food to go through and appear in the stools, with oliguria or haematuria . . .*'

(Zhangfu biaoben yongyao shi)

From the above it may be seen that the Chinese conception agrees to some extent with that of the West, particularly in regard to the digestive function of the small intestine. The Chinese consider however that the main part of the process of 'rotting and ripening' takes place in the stomach, while we in the West would probably consider the small intestine, with its many enzymes (enterokinase, lipase, amylase, sucrase, lactase, maltase, polypeptidases, alkaline phosphatase) to be of greater importance in this respect. This relative contradiction may be explained by the difference between the anatomical stomach, and what is felt on the pulse of the stomach by Chinese pulse diagnosis. As may be seen from their old drawings, the Chinese knew the anatomical position and configuration of the stomach. On pulse diagnosis, however, the pulse of the stomach also includes the first part of the duodenum, for duodenal ulcers show on the pulse of the stomach and not on that of the small intestine. Possibly for this reason the Chinese assign to the stomach some of the functions which we ascribe to the small intestine.

The idea that the small intestine divides the 'pure' from the 'impure', should be taken to mean that the 'impure' passes on from the small intestine to the large intestine as faeces, while the 'pure' is absorbed by the small intestine, and after having passed through the body, is excreted by the kidneys into the bladder as urine. Although this is not new to us, it does present the problem from an unaccustomed angle, from which we can derive new clinical insight, namely, that the small intestine controls the proportion of urine to faeces. Most of the water from the gastro-intestinal tract is absorbed in the small intestine—up to ten litres per day; the colon absorbs normally only 350 cc and the stomach minimal amounts in a day.

The Relationship between the Small Intestine and the Heart

This is the relationship of coupled organs, or as the Chinese say, mutually exterior and interior.

A red tongue with wasting of its substance belongs to heart fire, violent and abundant; together with this, however, there are often the symptoms of small quantities of dark urine, and sometimes there may be haematuria.

'*The heart controls blood and unites with the small intestine. If someone has a cardiac disease caused by heat, the heat will converge into the small intestine. Thus one will urinate blood.*'

(Chaoshi bingyuan)

With these conditions, if one uses the methods of purifying the heart and benefiting micturition, then one can cause the fire of the heart and small intestine to drain downwards with the urine.

A physiological relationship between the small intestine and heart, is far from obvious. There are nevertheless a few clues:—

In congestive cardiac failure, little urine is passed. This is supposed to be due to a reduced glomerular filtration, consequent on a diminished circulation. On the other hand the small intestinal absorption of water may perhaps play a part.

In the majority of fevers (fire disease), with tachycardia (fire symptom), the patient passes dark urine. The Chinese say this is due to the heart and small intestine; we would say it is due to dehydration and increased metabolism. This is not entirely contradictory for dehydration and increased metabolism are both fire symptoms.

Anatomically there is only a vague connection, in so far as in the embryo, the pericardial and peritoneal cavities intercommunicate via the pleural canal.

Symptomatology

Main Meridian Symptoms

Throat and pharynx ache, swelling below the jaw prevents the patient from turning his head, shoulders ache as though they are being pulled, upper arm hurts as though it were broken, deafness, tinnitus, area around ear becomes hot or cold, discolouration of the eyes, eyes water, cannot bend waist, abdomen distended, bradycardia.

SYMPTOMS OF EXCESS

Hyper-relaxation of joints, elbows useless.

SYMPTOMS OF INSUFFICIENCY

Formation of swellings or nodules.

Small Intestine Empty and Cold Symptoms

Urine colourless and in big quantities, oliguria, low abdominal pain, diarrhoea, borborygmi.
The pulse is fine and weak, the left pulse being extremely so.
The tongue is thinly furred white.

Small Intestine Full and Hot Symptoms

The navel and abdomen are swollen, only comfortable after flatus has been passed, small intestine painful. If severe then includes base of spine and texticles, urine dark, dysuria, sometimes alternately hot and cold. If excessively hot then an intestinal ulcer may form.
The pulse is slippery and rapid, the left pulse particularly so.
The tongue is thickly furred yellow, the sides and point of tongue may be red.

Connecting Meridian (Luo) Symptoms

SYMPTOMS OF EXCESS

Bones and joints flaccid and weak, elbow joint cannot move.

SYMPTOMS OF INSUFFICIENCY

Nodules between the fingers.

Muscle Meridian Symptoms

Pain, muscular spasm and dysfunction along the course of the muscle. meridian Tinnitus and pain in ear extending to the jaws. Weak eyesight.

Course of Meridians

Small Intestine Main Meridian

Principal Course

The meridian starts at the little finger at Si1, goes along the embryological posterior and inner surface of the arm, over the side of the neck and face, to end in front of the ear at Si19.

Special Details

The meridian begins at Si1 at the end of the little finger, goes up the arm and over the scapula (? from Si13 via B36 to Si14 and ? from Si14 via B11 to Si15) and thence to Gv14.

From Gv14 over the shoulder to S12.

From S12 down the chest to connect with the heart at Cv17. It penetrates the diaphragm to reach the stomach at Cv13 and Cv12, and continues downward to end at the small intestine, to which it belongs.

From S12 a branch goes over the throat and jaw to the outer corner of the eye, and then enters the ear, following the course Si16, Si17, G1, (?T22), Si19 to (?T20).

Another branch starts from the jaw just above Si17, going across the cheek to the inner corner of the eye at B1, and thence on to Si18.

Small Intestine Connecting Meridian (Luo)—Si7

The meridian begins above the wrist at Si7, ascending along the arm to the tip of the shoulder. It links with the heart Luo.

Small Intestine Muscle Meridian

The meridian begins at the end of the little finger, and unites at the wrist; ascends the forearm to unite on the medial side of the olecranon; ascends and unites posterior to the armpit. Goes over the shoulder to unite at the mastoid process, whence a branch enters the ear. Another branch continues over the ear and descends anteriorly to unite at the jaw; whence it ascends to the outer corner of the eye.

The original branch goes over the jaw in front of the ear to the outer corner of the eye, whence it ascends to the forehead and unites at the temple.

Small Intestine and Heart Divergent Meridians

Small Intestine Divergent Meridian

The small intestine divergent meridian leaves the small intestine main meridian behind the shoulder in the axilla, whence it moves across the chest to the heart and then down the abdomen to link with the small intestine.

Heart Divergent Meridian

The heart divergent meridian leaves the heart main meridian in the axilla; it goes to the heart to which it belongs, thereafter ascending the throat and face to the inner corner of the eye.

Important Points

Metal	Si1	
Water	Si2	
Wood	Si3	Tonification
Fire	Si5	Fire point of Yang Sovereign fire meridian
Earth	Si8	Sedation
Source	Si4	
Luo	Si7	
Xi	Si6	
Alarm	Cv4	
Associated	B27	

CHAPTER VIII

BLADDER

Traditional Chinese and Western Scientific Conceptions

The Bladder Controls the Storing of Fluid

'*The bladder is the official of a region, and fluid is stored in it.*'

(Su Wen, linglan midian lun)

In the above quotation fluid means urine. After food and drink have been turned into fluid (other meaning) by the stomach and spleen, this is transported to the whole body in order to nourish it. But the Fluid essential to the body has a normal level. The remainder, apart from a small part which is expelled to the exterior of the body as sweat, passes through the triple warmer water path, and is transported down to the bladder as urine.

'*Urine is the surplus of the body's fluid.*'

(Chaoshi bingyuan)

Therefore fluid, urine and sweat have a close relationship in waxing and waning, fullness and emptiness. If there is an excess of urine, then the fluid within the body will decrease; conversely, if sweating is excessive, or violent vomiting or diarrhoea cause the level of fluid to decrease, the volume of urine will also decrease, and in extreme cases there will be no micturition. Again, in hot weather there is much sweating, and therefore little micturition. In cold weather there is little sweating, but much micturition.

The Relationship between the Bladder and the Kidneys

The bladder (leg greater Yang meridian) and the kidney (leg lesser Yin meridian) have a reciprocal relationship of exterior and interior, *i.e.*, they are coupled meridians and organs.

'*The kidneys unite the bladder, the bladder is the Fu of Fluid.*'

(Ling Shu, benshu pian)

The ability of Fluid to become urine is also closely connected with the Qi transformation action of the kidneys.

'*The bladder is the official of a region, Fluid is stored in it; if the Qi moves, then one can urinate.*'

(Su Wan, linglan midian lun)

Thus, although retention and incontinence of urine are principally an abnormality of the bladder, sometimes deficiency of kidney Qi or deficiency of fire of destiny, can also produce these symptoms. In treatment, one should increase the kidney Qi or tonify the fire of destiny.

Case History. A male patient had to urinate about fifteen times a day. The pulse of the kidney and bladder were weak.

Stimulation at K5 made him better; stimulation at K3 made him worse. After twelve treatments he urinated four times a day.

Case History. A female patient suffered from headache and general fatigue over a period of many years. There were no bladder symptoms. Various points were stimulated, amongst them K5. This caused the patient 'to disappear behind every bush on the way home' to her house in the country, to the amusement of her friends in the car with her. This excessive urination stopped after one day, with the improvement of her headaches and fatigue. She was cured after repeated treatments.

It should be noted that in the first case history mentioned above K5 diminished bladder irritation, while in the second case history K5 increased bladder irritation.

General

The kidneys 'open the holes in the ears', control the loins and lumbar region, the sacral area, and to some extent the whole back. They also rule the bones. Therefore when the kidneys are diseased there are frequently symptoms in these areas.

Case History. A patient had mild tinnitus of four months' duration. The pulse of the kidney was weak.

Stimulation at K1 cured the condition. It should be noted though that tinnitus of longer duration (over six months) can only rarely be cured by acupuncture—unless it is catarrhal.

The Bladder, Associated Points and Metamerism

The bladder meridian differs from all others, as there are on it the associated points (Yu) of all other meridians. The associated points have a more or less segmental distribution, the only acupuncture points that have a distribution reminiscent of lower animals such as the earth worm, in which most structures are metamerically arranged.

In the human embryo the kidney is the only internal organ with a metameric arrangement similar to that of the associated points of the bladder. The pronephros, mesonephros and metanephros are of course kidneys and not bladders, but I think the function in the embryo is close enough for a comparison to be drawn; the external glomerulus of the pronephros opening into the coelonic cavity, for there is no bladder.

The pronephros originates from the 2nd to the 14th somite, the mesonephros from the 9th to the 26th, and the metanephros the 26th to 28th; *i.e.*, all the associated points alongside the vertebral column are within this range.

The bladder meridian probably goes along the back, as the pronephric duct runs dorsal to the nephrotome, between this and the ectoderm, to reach the cloaca.

Diseases along the Course of the Bladder Meridian

Points on the bladder meridian seem to have a greater effect on diseases of the spinal cord, than points on other meridians. Possibly this is because the bladder meridian runs paravertebrally, and a meridian always controls all structures in its neighbhourhood. In the embryo the nephrotome and the neural tube are likewise near one another.

Case Histories. I have treated several patients with disseminated sclerosis at an early stage of the disease, by stimulating point B62, or the paravertebral bladder points. The majority noticed a remarkable improvement within a few minutes or hours of treatment, the effect usually lasting several days. I do not think I have ever achieved a permanent improvement or cure, even with repeated treatments.

Haemorrhoids are likewise partially affected by the bladder meridian (see also the section on the liver), for the bladder meridian and meridian divergence run alongside the anus.

Certain types of occiptial neuralgia or pain at the medial end of the eyebrows may be cured by treating the bladder or kidney meridians. Care should be taken to differentiate these from the nearby gall bladder meridian.

Case History. A patient had unilateral supra-orbital neuralgia over the middle and medial part of the eyebrows. Stimulation of the liver at Liv8 on the opposite side removed the pain over the middle of the eyebrow —which had been in the region of and below point G14—within minutes. The pain at the medial end of the eyebrow—in the region of B2— remained, but was later removed by stimulating B60 on the same side.

Sciatica and lumbago may also be treated via the bladder meridian, in so far as the pain follows the distribution of this meridian. Sometimes points on the feet are best, sometimes those in the lumbar or sacral region. Choosing exactly the right point decides whether the patient will be cured in a few, or in many treatments, or even at all. Other types of lumbago or sciatica have to be treated via other meridians.

Symptomatology

Main Meridian Symptoms

Qi rushes upwards causing headache, pupils of eyes appear as though about to come out, nape of neck hurts as though being dragged and pulled, spine is painful, waist feels as if it is broken, lumbago, sciatica, hip joint cannot move, spasm of muscles in popliteal fossa calf and ankle, haemorrhoids, intermittent fevers, madness, insanity, yellowish discolouration of eyes, excessive lachrymation, clear or bloody nasal discharge.

SYMPTOMS OF EXCESS

Anosmia, headache, pain along spine.

SYMPTOMS OF INSUFFICIENCY

Epistaxis.

Bladder Full and Hot Symptoms

If damp and heat are congealed and bladder Qi transforms but does not motivate, then urine is passed in small quantities, is yellow-red in colour, is possibly turbid, and there is dysuria with a hot burning feeling during micturition and an abnormal smell; if severe there may be urinary incontinence and pain that is difficult to bear, the urine possibly being thick and bloody. There are also cases of a fusion of damp and heat, collecting to form a stone or gravel. Other organs may also influence micturition, for example, if damp and heat enter the bladder from the small intestine, the urine may become yellow-red, or there may be retention of urine.

Bladder Empty and Cold Symptoms

If the kidney Yang is deficient and there is a deficiency of the function of warming and transforming water and Qi, this may induce empty cold symptoms of the bladder, resulting in frequency of micturition, the urine being clear and light in colour, or in retention or urine, the face being blackish or oedematous. If the orthodox Qi is empty and weak, the bladder often loses its normal receiving action and causes incontinence of urine, or frequency of micturition. Although they are in the bladder, these diseases in fact concern the whole body, because the bladder is the Fu of the kidneys. The lungs also have the function of regulating water and Qi, therefore the disease signs are all the result of kidney Qi being deficient or lung Qi being weak.

Connecting Meridian (Luo) Symptoms

SYMPTOMS OF EXCESS

Clear nasal discharge, blocked nose, cold nose, pain in cervical spine.

SYMPTOMS OF INSUFFICIENCY

Clear nasal discharge, epistaxis.

Muscle Meridian Symptoms

Little toe and heel swollen and painful, cramp at back of knee, pain in back, muscular cramp at the back of the neck, inability to raise shoulders, upper arm and shoulder stiff and painful, inability to move shoulder girdle from side to side.

Course of Meridians

Bladder Main Meridian

Principal Course

The meridian starts at the inner corner of the eye at B1, then goes over the head to the neck, where it divides into two parallel meridians which rejoin at the buttock or the knee, according to interpretation. Thence it goes along the embryologically posterior and inner surface of the leg, to terminate at the little toe at B67.

Special Details

The meridian starts at the inner corner of the eye at B1, goes to B2, and thence via Gv24 to B3.

A branch goes from B7 (? via G7) to G8, G9, G10, G11, G12.

The main meridian, apart from going over the cranium along the course of the bladder meridian, also goes from B7 to Gv20, whence it enters the brain and emerges at the nape of the neck.

From B9 via Gv17 (? and Gv16) to B10.

From B10 via Gv14 (? and Gv13) to B11.

From B11 alongside the spinal column to B23, where it connects with the kidneys, and enters the bladder to which it belongs.

A branch continues downwards, making a zigzag on the inner surface of the buttocks to B50, and then goes down the thigh to B54.

Another branch leaves B10, going lateral to the main meridian to B49, thence via G30 it crosses the other branch between B51 and B52, to join it at B54.

From B54 it goes down the leg to end at the little toe at B67.

Bladder Connecting Meridian (Luo)—B58

This meridian begins above the ankle at B58 and links with the kidney meridian Luo.

Bladder Muscle Meridian

This meridian begins in the little toe, unites in the external malleolus; ascends and unites at the lateral corner of the popliteal fossa. From the external malleolus it goes to and unites in the heel; ascends the calf and unites at the back of the knee. The divergence from the external malleolus to the back of the knee unites in the calf. The main meridian muscle ascends to the buttocks where it unites; and then ascends para-vertebrally to the nape of the neck. A branch goes across the neck to unite in the root of the tongue. The main meridian muscle continues up to unite in the occiput; going over the cranium to unite in the nose. A branch arches over the eyebrows to unite over the cheek. A branch from the upper part of the shoulders goes to the tip of the shoulders where it unites. Another branch continues below the armpit to the supra-clavicular fossa where it ascends to unite over the mastoid process. Another branch from the supra-clavicular fossa ascends from the supra-clavicular fossa to unite in the cheek joining the circum-orbital branch.

Bladder and Kidney Divergent Meridians

Bladder Divergent Meridian

The bladder divergent meridian leaves the main bladder meridian behind the knee, whence it ascends the back of the thigh to the inferior gluteal fold where it divides into two. The one part goes to the bladder and then enters and is dispersed in the kidney. The other part ascends para-vertebrally to the heart, in which it is dispersed, and then continues to ascend to the nape of the neck, where it joins its parent main bladder meridian.

Kidney Divergent Meridian

The kidney divergent meridian leaves the kidney main meridian behind the knee, whence it ascends up the posterior surface of the thigh and then para-vertebrally to the kidney at the level of the 2nd lumbar vertebra. Here it is associated with the Dai mo and then ascends over the abdomen and thorax to link with the root of the tongue. Thereafter it passes laterally to the nape of the neck where it meets the bladder main meridian.

Important Points

Metal	B67	Tonification
Water	B66	Water point of Yang water meridian
Wood	B65	Sedation
Fire	B60	
Earth	B54	
Source	B64	
Luo	B58	
Xi	B63	
Alarm	Cv3	
Associated	B28	

CHAPTER IX

KIDNEY

Traditional Chinese and Western Scientific Conceptions

The Kidneys Store Jing

The kidneys store two types of Jing; firstly the Jing of the five Zang and six Fu, and secondly the Jing of reproduction.

The Jing of the Zang and Fu originates from the ingested water and food; it is a basic nourishing substance which maintains the life and movement of the body. It is stored in the kidneys and is distributed from there to the rest of the body when required.

'*The kidneys control water, receive the Jing of the Zang and Fu and store it.*'

(Su Wen, shango tianzhen lun)

The Jing of reproduction is the Jing of sexual fertilisation possessed by both male and female; it is the basic substance which enables man to reproduce. From the time of conception to birth the Jing Qi is in abundance and is able to nourish the embryo.

This type of Jing is formed from the transformation of the combined kidney Qi of Former Heaven (pre-natal) and the Jing Qi of the five Zang of Latter Heaven (post-natal), and it is stored in the kidney. The development and decline of Jing is controlled by the kidneys; hence diseases such as spermatorrhoea, nocturnal emissions, deficiency of semen or infertility, are all controlled by the kidneys.

Case History. A man in his forties had become impotent during the previous year. He also had slight lumbago.

He was cured by stimulating K5 and Gv4. (Governing vessel points in the lumbar and sacral area have an effect on the kidney.)

The Relationship between Kidney Qi and Birth and Growth

Kidney Qi is endowed with the Jing Qi of the Former Heaven of the mother and father. After the mother has become pregnant it is the basis for the development of the foetus. After birth the kidney Qi is nourished by the Jing Qi of water and food, and is thus able to promote the growth of the body.

'*When a female reaches the age of 7 the kidney Qi is abundant, the teeth change and the hair grows long. At the age of 14 menstruation arrives, the vessel of conception communicates, the Dai mo and the Chong mo are abundant, menstruation occurs at the proper time, therefore there are children. At 21 the kidney Qi is balanced, thus the true teeth grow and develop. . . . At 49 the vessel of conception is empty, the Dai mo and Chong mo are decayed and small, menstruation is exhausted, the Dao (Tao or Path) of earth does not penetrate, therefore form is destroyed and there are no children.*'

'*When a man reaches the age of 8 the kidney Qi is full, the teeth change and the hair grows long. At the age of 16 the kidney Qi is abundant, sexual substance (Tienkui occurs in males and females) arrives, Jing Qi flows out, Yin and Yang harmonise, therefore it is possible to have children. At 24 the kidney Qi is balanced, and muscles and bones are strong, therefore true teeth grow and develop; . . . At 40 the kidney Qi decays, the teeth wither and the hair falls; . . . At 56 the liver Qi decays, the muscles cannot move, sexual substance is exhausted, there is little Jing, the kidney Zang decays, form and substance are all at their limits. At 64 the teeth and hair have gone. . . . Now that the five Zang are decayed, the muscles and bones have decayed, sexual substance is finished; therefore the hair becomes white, the body is heavy, walking is not upright and there are no children.*'

'*If people have children in old age this means that their normal span of life exceeds the normal limits, their Qi and blood vessels continue to penetrate normally, and the kidney Qi has a surplus.*'

(Su Wen, shango tian zhen lun)

From the above quotations it can be seen that sexual ability and production of Jing, together with the growing processes of the whole body, are closely connected with the kidneys. Thus there is a saying: 'The kidneys are the root of Former Heaven.'

Case History. A woman of thirty had tried to become pregnant for five years. Tubal insufflation and the normal gynaecological tests were negative. Hormones and psychiatry had failed. She had slight lumbago, was slightly tense during intercourse and the kidney pulse was weak.

She was stimulated at K5 and several ancillary points, and became pregnant within one month. The tension during intercourse had also stopped but the lumbago remained.

The Kidneys Control the Fire of the Gate of Life

The fire of the Gate of Life is also called Minister Fire. The Gate of Life has the meaning of "the basis of life". Minister Fire is spoken of in referring to the Sovereign Fire controlled by the heart, and has the function of benefiting the Sovereign Fire. The kidney Zang controls water and stores Jing, and also controls the fire of the Gate of Life, and is the dwelling place of the original Yin and original Yang Qi (also called true Yin, true Yang or kidney Yin and kidney Yang). As a consequence all the functioning of the Zang and growth, together with conception and birth, all depend on the mutual assistance of kidney water, and fire of destiny.

'*The Gate of Life is the sea of Jing and blood; spleen and stomach are the sea of water and nourishment; together they are the root of the five Zang and six Fu. Moreover the Gate of Life is the origin of original Qi and the dwelling place of water and fire; without this the Yin Qi of the five Zang cannot nourish and the Yang Qi of the five Zang cannot begin. The spleen and stomach use the earth of the middle region, and without fire they cannot create. . . . The spleen and stomach are the root of irrigation and obtain the Qi of Latter Heaven; the Gate of Life is the source of transformation and obtains the Qi of Former Heaven.*'

'*The Gate of Life has the strength of fire, called original Yang, and this is the fire of living things.*'

(Jingyue quanshu)

The above view can be applied pathologically. In a person whose kidney Yin is deficient the deficiency may produce the Empty Yang Violent Above symptoms of dizziness in the head and eyes, caused by liver Yin being deficient. Alternatively, kidney Yin deficiency can cause the heart Yin to be deficient, producing heart Fire Violent and Vigorous symptoms such as palpitations, insomnia, etc. In severe cases it may cause the lung Yin to be deficient, producing the symptoms of dry cough, haemoptysis and spontaneous sweating.

Case History. A patient had palpitations for no apparent reason and had suffered from insomnia over a period of two years.

Pulse diagnosis showed an underactivity of the kidney and not an overactivity of the heart as expected.

Stimulation at K2 cured the condition.

Deficiency of kidney Yang may cause spleen Yang to be deficient, producing various types of diarrhoea. Or it may cause heart Qi to be empty and weak causing palpitations. In severe cases it results in an emptiness and weakness of lung Qi and produces dyspnoea and Yang empty with spontaneous sweating.

In all these cases one must nourish the kidney Yin or stimulate the kidney fire. On the other hand if the fire of the Gate of Life is deficient, this can cause a decrease of sexual desire or even impotence; conversely, if the minister fire is moving recklessly this can cause excessive sexual desire. In the first case one must warm and tonify the kidney Yang, and in the second strengthen water to regulate fire. This is consistant with the view that the fire of the Gate of Life of the kidney Zang is directly related to the function of reproduction.

The Kidneys Control the Bone and Marrow and Communicate with the Brain

The growth and development of the bones and marrow have a definite connection with the kidneys; for example the Su Wen recognises that 'bone paralysis disease' is due to 'kidney Qi hot'. When the kidneys receive heat which injures the kidney Yin, this causes the bones to wither and the marrow to decline, so that the loins and back cannot move and turn, and both legs are paralysed and wasted, and one cannot stand up straight.

'*The kidneys create bone and marrow.*'

(Su Wen, yinyang yingziang dalun)

'*If the kidneys do not create then the marrow cannot be full.*'

(Su Wen, nitiao lun)

The meeting and unifying of the marrow is in the brain.

'*The brain is the sea of marrow.*'

(Ling Shu, hailun)

'*All marrow belongs to the brain.*'

(Su Wen, wuzang shengcheng lun)

Since the brain is the meeting point of all marrow, and marrow is also formed by transformation of the kidney Jing, the kidney Zang is not only the basis of the Zang and Fu, but is also connected to the functioning of the bones, marrow and brain.

'*The kidneys are the official who does energetic work and excels by his ability and cleverness.*'

(Su Wen, linglan midian lun)

Thus if the kidneys are strong and full, then the Jing strength of the body is full and copious, physical energy is great, and at the same time the brain feels that it is strong, is clever and able. On the other hand if the kidney Qi is deficient, not only can it cause aching loins and painful bones, along with body weakness, but so also can it cause amnesia, insomnia, mental confusion, tinnitus, etc. To cure all these conditions one must tonify the kidneys to increase Jing and restore the kidney Qi.

Case History. A ten-year-old boy was near the bottom of his class. Previously he had been reasonably bright, but now his mind wandered and he was unable to concentrate.

He was cured after two treatments at K8.

This type of disturbance can only be cured if it is physiological. If the boy's laziness were due to his innate nature or to faulty upbringing, it would not have been cured by acupuncture. An astute clinical judgement is required to differentiate these different types, so as to decide which may be successfully treated.

The Kidneys Open the Holes in the Ears and the Two Yin

In the upper part of the body the kidneys open the holes in the ears, in the lower part they open the front and rear Yin (urethra and anus).

'*The kidney Qi penetrates to the ears; if the kidney is harmonious then the five sounds can be heard.*'

(Ling Shu, modu pian)

Clinically this means that those with an empty kidney often have tinnitus, in severe cases deafness; in early cases this may be treated by tonifying the kidneys.

The opening of the two Yin holes means chiefly the connection between the kidneys with micturition on the one hand and defaecation on the other; the kidneys are the water Zang and thus have the function of managing all the fluid in the body. This function however requires the collaboration of both kidney water and kidney fire, *i.e.*, the fire of the Gate of Life. Thus the correct functioning of micturition and defaecation, although related to the spleen, stomach, large intestine, bladder, etc., is also related to the fire of the Gate of Life. If kidney water is deficient it may cause dry stools and constipation or oliguria. If the fire of the Gate of Life is deficient it may cause diarrhoea, urinary incontinence or polyuria. If the kidney Zang's function is abnormal, Qi does not transform water, and this may cause the fluids to remain inside the body, causing retention of urine, oedema and ascites.

'*The kidney is the gateway to the stomach; if the gateway is not functioning, water accumulates and acts according to its class. Above and below it overflows into the skin and causes swelling.*'

(Su Wen, shuirexue lun)

This type of water retention caused by the kidney's loss of normal function may often be treated by stimulating the kidney Yin and kidney Yang.

Case History. A patient thought there might be something wrong as she urinated only twice a day. She also had extreme fatigue which nearly made me think of Addison's disease. (Kidney and adrenal cortex are related in acupuncture.)

The fatigue was reduced and the urination increased to nearer normal frequency by treatment of a large number of acupuncture points for a long time, using mainly kidney points.

The Kidneys, Adrenal Cortex and Gonads

The majority of diseases of the kidneys, adrenal cortex or gonads, are revealed by pulse diagnosis at the pulse of the kidney. If an underactivity of the pulse is found at this position, no more can be told than that there is a disturbance which has its most probable seat in one or other of these three organs. Further elucidation of the history or examination is required to differentiate the one affected.

I think the best explanation for the close relationship between these three organs lies in embryology, for all are derived, at least partially, from the urogenital ridge:

The testis is formed from the urogenital ridge, utilising both the pronephric duct and mesonephric tubules as excretory duct.

The ovary is likewise formed from the urogenital ridge. Its excretory duct of Müller is induced to arise by the presence of the pronephric duct, not forming if this is absent. In sharks the Müllerian duct arises by a longitudinal splitting of the pronephric duct.

The adrenal cortex also arises from the urogenital ridge, dorsal and medial to the gonad. The medulla arises separately from the same tissues as the sympathetic. Abberant adrenals may accompany the gonads or may be found buried within the kidneys.

The definitive mammalian kidney, the metanephros, is formed partly (ureter, renal pelvis, calyces, collecting tubules) from the pronephric or mesonephric duct, and partly from the nephrogenic cord (secretory tubules and Bowman's capsule), a specialisation of the urogenetial fold.

The above close embryological inter-relationship between the kidneys, adrenal cortex and gonads, is also reflected in their physiological function:

The adrenal cortex not only produces the cortisone-like hormones but also (*a*) the sex hormones—androgens, oestrogens and progesterone, and (*b*) influences water metabolism with either retention of urine or an excessive diuresis.

The sexual (gonad) effect of hyperadrenocortism, especially if due to a tumour, may be seen in the foetus as a pseudohermaphrodite, in prepubertal boys as pubertus praecox, in girls and women as masculinisation, and in the adult male as adrenal feminism.

The pulse diagnosis seems to record the primitive condition, that is when all three organs and functions were probably more or less the same.

The Kidneys and Bones

The bones, particularly the vertebral column, seem to be dependent on the kidney—or what might be called the kidney complex.

Any disturbance in the lumbar or sacral area is always found in the pulse of the kidney and bladder. This can perhaps be partly explained by the dorsal position of the kidneys and the close connection between the developing metanephros and the notochord.

From the above an association between the parathyroids and the kidney would be expected. This is in fact the case, as hyperparathyroidism with acidosis and phosphate retention, may be caused by advanced renal disease. Likewise hypoparathyroidism may be caused by chronic nephritis. The reverse may also be seen as primary hyperparathyroidism may cause nephrocalcinosis. Primary hypoparathyroidism though has no obvious renal symptoms. The above are of course advanced pathological states, but I am sure that investigation would show that the stimulation of points on the kidney meridian influences the production and circulation of parathormone.

Symptomatology

Main Meridian Symptoms

Hungry and yet no appetite for food, dark complexion like lacquered ash, rusty sputum, severe dyspnoea, wishing to stand when sitting and then the eyes blur as if blind, vision blurred, fondness for lying down and sleeping, frightened, nocturnal enuresis, hot lips, hot dry tongue, swollen pharynx, heart and chest feel oppressed, palpitations, heart suspended as though hungry, jaundice, abdominal distension, diarrhoea, bones ache, difficulty in walking, soles of feet hot and painful, extremely cold.

SYMPTOMS OF EXCESS

Intestinal blockage?, depression.

SYMPTOMS OF INSUFFICIENCY

Lumbago, sciatica.

Kidney Empty Symptoms

In kidney diseases the principal symptoms if Yin is empty, are spermatorrhoea, tinnitus, dental neuralgia, lumbago, sciatica, weakness and aching of the legs; if the condition is severe there can be paralysis.

At times this may affect other organs.

If kidney Yin is deficient and liver fire becomes vigorous and abundant, there will be: dry mouth, dry throat, dizziness in head and eyes, red face and ears, ears with a noise in them similar to that when covered by a sea-shell, also deafness.

If the lungs are affected then there may be coughing, night sweats, haemoptysis and emaciation. This is caused by deficient Yin and vigorous fire, which ascends and burns the lung metal.

Kidney and Heart

The kidneys belong to water, the heart belongs to fire, water and fire must contend. If kidney Yin is empty and heart fire blazes upwards, this can cause the Shen in the heart to be ill at ease, causing insomnia, etc. Conversely, if the heart Shen is ill at ease, or if Shen Qi is decayed and weak, this easily becomes a kidney disease, causing spermatorrhoea, tinnitus and lumbago.

Kidney Yang Empty Symptoms

If the kidney Yang is empty then Jing Qi cannot collect, and there is always Jing cold slippery leakage, *i.e.*, involuntary loss of seminal fluid, impotence, feeling of cold in waist and legs, numb and weak feet. If kidney Yang is deficient and cannot transform water, this can cause the water Qi to remain collected in the body, causing oliguria and pale lips; if the condition is severe there may be superficial oedema, heaviness of the body and ascites. Apart from this, the five types of diarrhoea are due to the kidney Yang being too empty and weak to warm and move the spleen Earth, thus causing diminution of the spleen's functions of transporting and transforming water and Qi, and of moving and transforming food and drink. Other symptoms caused by kidney Yang being empty and not being able to disseminate water fluid, include dryness of the mouth associated with drinking of much fluid, increased micturition, and a desire to urinate immediately after drinking. If the kidneys are empty and cannot receive Qi, then Qi rebels and escapes upwards producing numb and cold feet and Qi rebellious dyspnoea. If the condition is severe there is perspiration of the forehead and the pulse is deep, and there is oedema of the feet, in which case the disease has already become dangerous.

Connecting Meridian (Luo) Symptoms

SYMPTOMS OF EXCESS

Feeling of depression in the region of the heart, oliguria, constiptation.

SYMPTOMS OF INSUFFICIENCY

Pain at the waist.

Muscle Meridian Symptoms

Spasm or pain in the sole of the foot and those places passed by the muscle meridian. There may also be epilepsy, convulsions and generalised muscular spasms. If the disease occurs posteriorly the patient cannot bend forward. If it occurs anteriorly the patient cannot lean back or look up, *i.e.*, if the Yang is diseased there is difficulty in flexion, if the Yin is diseased there is difficulty in extension.

Course of Meridians

Kidney Main Meridian

Principal Course

The meridian starts on the sole of the foot at K1, goes up the embryologically anterior and inner surface of the leg, over the abdomen and chest near the midline, to end near the sterno-clavicular joint at K27.

Special Details

The meridian begins under the little toe and then goes to K1. (According to some descriptions the points round the internal malleolus are in the following order: K2, K3, K4, K5, K6, K7.

In other books K2, K6, K5, K4, K3, K7. Occasionally there are other variations.)

From K8 to Sp6 to K9.

From the inside of the thigh, the main meridian goes to Gv1, then up the spine to the kidneys to which it belongs, thereafter connecting with the bladder.

From the bladder it goes to Cv4, Cv3, K11 and thence over the abdomen and chest to K27.

The direct meridian goes from the kidney through the liver and diaphragm to ramify in the lungs, whence it follows the trachea to enter the root of the tongue.

From the lungs a branch goes to the heart, spreads over the chest, thence going to Cv17. This branch joins the circulation-sex meridian, which may be taken to be the branch from K22 to Cx1.

Kidney Connecting Meridian (Luo)—K6

The meridian begins at the ankle at K6, and ascends with the meridian to the pericardium and thence penetrates to the back. It links with the bladder meridian Luo.

Kidney Muscle Meridian

The meridian begins under the little toe, follows the course of the spleen meridian for a short part of the foot, and then unites at the heel; ascends the lower leg and unites at the medial corner of the popliteal fossa where it meets the bladder muscle meridian; ascends the inner side of the thigh together with the spleen muscle meridian to unite at the genitalia; ascends the spine to unite at the occiput where it meets the bladder muscle meridian.

Important Points

Wood	K1	Sedation
Fire	K2	
Earth	K5	
Metal	K7	Tonification
Water	K10	Water point of Yin water meridian
Source	K5	
Luo	K6	
Xi	K4	
Alarm	G25	
Associated	B23	

CHAPTER X

CIRCULATION-SEX

(Envelope of the Heart or Pericardium)

Traditional Chinese and Western Scientific Conceptions

The Chinese characters for this meridian mean, literally, 'envelope of the heart'. In modern Chinese the same characters are used to denote the pericardium, something which was not known in the early days of acupuncture. I have used the word circulation-sex, as it is used by several other European doctors. The function of the meridian is partially concerned with the circulation. However the pulse position of this meridian (3rd position right deep) represents both this meridian and the kidney meridian, particularly the Mingmen, which is concerned with the sexual function of the kidney. Hence the name circulation-sex.

This meridian is the external protector of the heart and has the function of guarding the heart Zang. At the same time it has the function of administering the controlling action of the heart.

'*The pericardium is the organ from which the feeling of happiness comes.*'

(Su Wen, linglan midian lun)

'*The heart is the great controller of the Zang and Fu . . . if an evil enters the heart it will injure it as the heart cannot withstand it; if the heart is injured then the Shen will leave and if the Shen leaves then one will die. Thus the presence of evil in the heart depends on the pericardium.*'

(Ling Shu, xieke pian)

Thus it was recognised that the pericardium can receive evils on behalf of the heart. For example, symptoms such as confused Shen, trismus, incoherent speech, etc., are all 'evil entering the pericardium', and from the point of view of treatment one uses the method of purifying the heart and sedating fire, or purifying the heart and pacifying Shen.

Case History. A patient in her thirties had recurrent bouts of severe depression, during several of which she had unsuccessfully tried to commit suicide. She thought the cause of her depressions lay in her upbringing as a child, which involved more abstract psychology than common sense. During the previous fifteen years she had visited many psychiatrists and had tried several drugs—both of which had helped, though only to a minimal extent.

Chinese pulse diagnosis and symptomatology were inconclusive at least to me. The first four treatments, during which several meridians were used, had no effect. The fifth treatment in which I stimulated the circulation-sex meridian at Cx7 for the first time, caused her to feel nearly normal by the next day, the cure being complete with one further treatment. As this was a long standing history, a few booster treatments were required for a further two years to prevent recurrence.

What is precisely governed by this (and the triple warmer) meridian is less specifically stated in Chinese texts than the influence of the other ten meridians. Clinically it is also harder to define its effect in terms of understandable anatomy or physiology. Amongst its functions are cardiac, circulatory, renal and mental.

The pericardium itself seems hardly worth considering amongst the important organs, though it should be remembered that in the human embryo the pericardium is as big as the head and is separated from it only by the pharyngeal membrane. Presumably the size of an organ has at least a little to do with its importance.

Symptomatology

Main Meridian Symptoms

Heart feels hot, forearm and elbow stiffen and feel constrained, axilla becomes swollen, chest and ribs feel oppressed, thumping and lurching of the heart, cardiac pain going into throat, face flushed, pyrexia, vision blurred, eyes discoloured, wild laughter without ceasing, hot palm of hand.

SYMPTOMS OF EXCESS

Cardiac pain.

SYMPTOMS OF INSUFFICIENCY

Head and neck stiff.

I have not been able to find in Chinese texts a systematic classification into HOT, COLD, FULL, EMPTY, as for the other meridians. These may though be calculated from basic principles.

Connecting Meridian (Luo) Symptoms

SYMPTOMS OF EXCESS
Painful heart.

SYMPTOMS OF INSUFFICIENCY
Stiffness and inability to turn the head.

Muscle Meridian Symptoms
Muscular spasm, pain and dysfunction along the course of the meridian. Haemoptysis with pain in the chest.

Course of Meridians

Circulation-Sex Main Meridian

Principal Course
Starting lateral to the nipple at Cx1, the meridian arches over the axilla, to go down the middle of the anterior surface of the arm between the other two arm Yin meridians and ends at the middle finger at Cx9.

Special Details
The meridian begins in the middle of the chest, emerging from the pericardium to which it belongs, and represented by Cv17. It penetrates the diaphragm and passes through the abdomen being connected with the upper middle and lower divisions of the triple warmer; this part of its course is represented by the points Cv12 and Cv7.

A branch from Cv17 goes across the chest to Cx1 and thence down the arm to Cx9.

A branch leaves Cx8 to go to T1.

Circulation-Sex Connecting Meridian (Luo)—Cx6
The meridian begins above the wrist at Cx6 and ascends with its meridian. Links with the circulation-sex meridian Luo.

Circulation-Sex Muscle Meridian
The meridian begins at the middle finger and goes up the forearm to unite at the elbow; continuing along the upper arm to unite below

the armpit; thereafter dispersing through the front and back of the chest.

A branch from the axilla disperses in the chest and unites at the cardia.

Important Points

Wood	Cx9	Tonification
Fire	Cx8	Fire point of Yin Ministerial fire meridian
Earth	Cx7	Sedation
Metal	Cx5	
Water	Cx3	
Source	Cx7	
Luo	Cx6	
Xi	Cx4	
Alarm	?Cv17 or ?Cv15	
Associated	B14	

CHAPTER XI

TRIPLE WARMER

Traditional Chinese and Western Scientific Conceptions

The Division of the Three Warmers According to their Position

The Triple Warmer is one of the six Fu, but there are differences between it and the other Fu. The body is divided into the Upper Warmer, the Middle Warmer, and the Lower Warmer. From the cardia of the stomach to the base of the tongue, including the chest, and in particular the heart and lungs, is the region of the Upper Warmer. From the cardia to the pylorus of the stomach, including the upper abdomen, and in particular the spleen and stomach, is the region of the Middle Warmer. From the pylorus to the two Yin (urethra and anus), including the lower abdomen and in particular the liver, kidneys, large and small intestines and bladder, is the region of the Lower Warmer.

'*The Upper Warmer, from the lower diaphragm below the heart to the upper orifice of the stomach controls receiving and does not expel. The Middle Warmer, at the middle of the stomach, has a middle position, controls the rotting and ripening of food and water. The Lower Warmer, at the upper orifice of the bladder, controls the division of the pure and impure, controls expelling and not receiving in order to transmit.*'

(Nanjing sanshiyinan shuo)

The Functional Division of the Triple Warmer

In general terms the function of the Triple Warmer is to circulate Qi blood and fluid, to rot and ripen food and water, and to harmonise the digestion of solid and liquid food.

'*Water and food enter through the mouth; they have five tastes; each one flowing into its own sea; the fluids all move along their own paths; therefore the three Warmers emit Qi in order to warm the flesh; that which fills the skin is Jin, that which remains and does not move is Ye.*'

(Ling Shu, wulong jinyue bielun)

'*The Triple Warmer is the path of water and food, the beginning and end of Qi.*'

(Nanjing, sanshiyinan)

The above quotations explain that the function of the Triple Warmer is to cause the Qi, blood and fluid which come from water and food to circulate in the skin and flesh and between the Zang and Fu; the stomach and spleen on the one hand and the Middle Warmer on the other (both are in the same region) control the rotting and ripening of water and food.

'*The Triple Warmer is the middle draining Fu and the digestion comes from this. It belongs to the bladder.*'

(Ling Shu, benshu pian)

Thus the Triple Warmer also has the function of clearing the digestive tract. However, the functions of the separate warmers are in control of specific things, and are closely associated with the organs which they include.

Upper Warmer

'*The Upper Warmer is like mist (fog, mist, vapour etc.).*'

(Ling Shu, yingwei shenghui pian)

This means that the upper warmer is described as having much Qi (the lungs control Qi, the chest is the sea of Qi) and its function is similar to mist in its all pervading irrigation. The Qi of the Upper Warmer originates in the Middle Warmer.

'*The Upper Warmer is a prime mover, it distributes the five food tastes, vapourises into the skin, fills the body, moistens the hair on the body, is like the irrigation of mist and dew, and is called Qi.*'

(Ling Shu, jueqi pian)

'*The spleen scatters Jing, Qi is like a cloud, a mist, and returns to the lungs. This is called Upper Warmer like mist.*'

(Zhangshi leijing)

The Upper Warmer's function of circulating Qi around the whole body and moistening and vapourising the skin, filling the body, moistening the hair and the exterior skin of the body, obtains nourishment and so develops the function of protecting the outside—a function which is called Wei Qi. If the Upper Warmer loses its normal function, the circulation becomes blocked, the skin and the space between the skin and flesh cannot obtain the warmth of Wei Qi, the opening and closing of the sweat holes (pores) is not effective, and thus may produce the symptoms of cold or fever. Apart from this the Upper Warmer also has the function of 'controlling reception'. The so-called reception includes both that of air and food and drink. Because the lungs (which control breathing) and the stomach (which controls the receiving of food and water) both operate in (literally 'open holes in') the Upper Warmer, the Upper Warmer is said to have the function of 'controlling reception.'

Middle Warmer

'*The Middle Warmer is like foam (froth, foam, bubbles etc.).*'
(Ling Shu, yingwei shenghui pian)

This refers to the appearance of the food and drink that has been transformed by the spleen and stomach. From the point of view of the scope of the Middle Warmer and the function of the Zang and Fu, which it includes, the most important aspects are the moving and transforming of water and food and the distilling of Qi, blood and fluid, which then nourish the whole body. Within this process, the power of transformation and movement includes the functions of the spleen and stomach and also the Lower Warmer.

'*The Middle Warmer also unites the middle of the stomach, and the Qi which is received there flushes the dregs, distils the fluid, transforms its essential and fine parts, and pours upwards into the lung meridian which then transforms it into blood.*'
(Ling Shu, yingwei shenghui pian)

'*The Middle Warmer receives Qi, extracts the juice and changes it into a substance. This is called blood.*'
(Ling Shu, jueqi pian)

Thus the function of the Middle Warmer is principally to take water and food and transform it into Qi blood and fluid, all of which have the function of nourishing. The Middle Warmer's attribute of being 'like foam' is the result of its physiological movement of 'changing, transforming, distilling the flushing'. If the action of the Middle Warmer is blocked it will harm the process of digestion and the transformation of Qi and blood.

Lower Warmer

'*The Lower Warmer is like a drain.*'
(Ling Shu, yingwei shenghui pian)

'*Drain means the flowing and draining of water. The Lower Warmer controls emitting and not receiving, departing and not returning.*'
(Zhangshi leijing)

Thus the principal function of the Lower Warmer is the draining and flushing of the pure and impure, and also the expulsion of urine and faeces.

'*The Lower Warmer helps the function of separation and passes the dregs into the large intestine.*'

'*The Lower Warmer permeates the fluid, unites with the bladder, controls emitting and not entering, divides pure and impure.*'

One type of diarrhoea is due to the pure and the impure not being separated, with retention or incontinence of urine, the bladder Qi having lost its function. This may be due to a dysfunction of the Lower Warmer.

The Relationship between the Triple Warmer and the Pericardium

The Triple Warmer and the pericardium are coupled meridians. In Chinese parlance they have an exterior and interior mutual relationship.

'*The Triple Warmer is the external protector of the Zang and Fu, the pericardium is the external protector of the heart, like the great walls of the Imperial Palace; thus both belong to Yang, and both are called Minister Fire. Moreover the meridians communicate reciprocally and are mutually exterior and interior.*'

(Zhangshi leijing)

In the above context the pericardium is called Yang because it protects the heart, taking upon itself diseases which would otherwise affect the heart; thus it is like the wall protecting the Imperial Palace. In the interior-exterior relationship of Triple Warmer and pericardium, however, the pericardium is Yin.

The heart and small intestine are called Sovereign Fire (or sometimes Princely Fire) while the pericardium and Triple Warmer are called Minister Fire, because the Minister protects the Sovereign. In other words the triple warmer and pericardium have protective functions, protecting on the one hand the Zang and the Fu in general, and on the other hand the heart.

Case History. A patient was excessively tired, so tired that she usually returned to bed again after breakfast. Her skin was hot, the superficial veins were always dilated, she had migraine and was nervous. TI cured her fatigue.

Symptomatology

Main Meridian Symptoms

Deafness, confused mind, pharyngitis, swollen jaws, pain in outer corner of eye, pain behind the ear and over mastoid, perspiring for no reason, distension of lower abdominal, inability to urinate, pain or loss of function along course of meridian.

SYMPTOMS OF EXCESS

Elbow in position of flexion.

SYMPTOMS OF INSUFFICIENCY

Elbow cannot be flexed.

Upper Warmer Symptoms

Includes principally the arm greater Yin lung meridian and the arm absolute Yin pericardium meridian.

The symptoms of the lung meridian are:—headache, slight dislike of wind and cold, body hot and spontaneous sweating, thirst, and possibly coughing with absence of thirst.

The pulse is neither slowed down nor tight, but moving and rapid.

If the condition is transmitted to the pericardium meridian, then the tongue is deep red, and there is agitation and thirst. If the condition is severe then the Shen is confused, causing incoherent speech, restless sleep, stiff tongue and cold limbs.

Middle Warmer Symptoms

Includes principally the leg Yang Ming stomach meridian and the leg greater Yin spleen meridian. Yang Ming controls dryness and the greater Yin controls damp.

The symptoms of the stomach meridian are:—no dislike of cold but dislike of heat, more severe in the afternoon, sweating, face and eyes red, harsh breathing, dense stools, dysuria, dry mouth and thirsty.

The pulse is large.

The tongue is furred old-yellow; if the condition is severe, it may be black and prickly.

The symptoms of the spleen meridian are:—moderate sensation of heat, comparatively heavy feeling after noon, mental dullness, head feels swollen and body heavy, melancholy feeling in chest and no appetite, dislike of all food and wish to vomit, micturition infrequent, defaecation sluggish, stools possibly very loose.

The pulse is slowed down.

The tongue has white and greasy fur.

Lower Warmer Symptoms

Includes principally the leg lesser Yin kidney meridian and the leg absolute Yin liver meridian. If the disease has reached this stage, then the fluid has withered and dried up.

The symptoms of the former (kidney) are:—comparative peace during day but agitation during night, dry mouth and no wish to drink, painful throat, inability to speak because of ulcers, the heart is agitated, oliguria, reddish urine.

The symptoms of the latter (liver) are:—alternating feelings of cold and heat, painful and hot heart, misery and melancholy, sometimes dry vomiting, perhaps headache and vomiting of saliva, heart feels hungry but unable to eat, emotions sometimes extremely depressed. If the symptoms are in upper part of body the mouth is dry and feels rotten; if in lower part of body then there may be diarrhoea and heaviness in rectum, perhaps wind-moving convulsions with feeling of cold, contracted testicles and painful abdomen, deafness.

Connecting Meridian (Luo) Symptoms

SYMPTOMS OF EXCESS

Restriction in movement of elbow joint.

SYMPTOMS OF INSUFFICIENCY

Elbow joint too flaccid, over-relaxed.

Muscle Meridian Symptoms

Muscular spasm, pain or dysfunction along the course of the meridian muscle.

Course of Meridians

Triple Warmer Main Meridian

Principal Course

The meridian starts at the end of the 4th finger at T1, goes up the posterior surface of the arm between the two other Yang meridians of the arms; thence it goes across the shoulders and neck, behind the ear, and over the face, to end at the lateral corner of the eyebrows at T23.

Special Details

The meridian begins at T1 at the tip of the 4th finger and goes up the arm to the shoulder at T14.

(? From T14 via Si12 to T15).

From T15 to G21, and over the shoulder to S12.

From here it descends to spread through the chest and is connected with the pericardium, going from S12 (?via Cx1) to Cv17.

From Cv17 it penetrates the diaphragm and goes to the three divisions of the triple warmer to which it belongs, represented by Cv17, Cv12 and Cv7.

A branch leaves S12 and goes (? via B11) to Gv14. From Gv14 to T16, T17, T18, T19, T20.

From T20 (? via G6) to G5, G4, G14, B1 down the naso-labial groove and lower jaw, to curl up the middle of the cheek and end at Si18. (Or possibly from T20 via an S shaped course to the eye at B1.)

From T17 a branch enters the ear to emerge in front of it at Si19, and thence goes via T21, T22 and T23 to end at G1. If the previously mentioned branch goes directly from T20 to B1, then this branch goes from T22 looping round the jaw, to Si18 and G1, to end at T23.

(? From T16 to G20 to G11.)

Triple Warmer Connecting Meridian (Luo)—T5

The meridian begins above the wrist at T5, goes up the outer surface of the arm and floods the chest. It links with the circulation-sex meridian Luo.

Triple Warmer Muscle Meridian

The meridian begins at the end of the fourth finger, unites at the wrist; goes up the forearm, unites at the elbow; ascends the upper arm goes over the shoulder, to the neck where it meets the small intestine muscle meridian. A branch goes to the jaw and links with the root of the tongue. The main muscle meridian ascends past the teeth to the ear, and then moves laterally to the outer corner of the eyes, whence it goes to the upper part of the temple, where it unites.

Triple Warmer and Circulation-Sex Divergent Meridians

Triple Warmer Divergent Meridian

The triple warmer divergent meridian leaves the triple warmer main meridian at the shoulder. One part goes to the crown of the head; the other part leaves the supra-clavicular fossa to disperse through the three divisions of the triple warmer in the chest and abdomen.

Circulation-Sex Divergent Meridian

The circulation-sex divergent meridian leaves the circulation-sex main meridian a little below the axilla. It enters the chest where it divides, the one part following the course of the triple warmer divergent meridian into the abdomen the other going to the throat, and thence behind the ear, where it meets the triple warmer meridian over the mastoid process.

Important Points

Metal	T1	
Water	T2	
Wood	T3	Tonification
Fire	T6	Fire point of Yang Ministerial fire meridian
Earth	T10	Sedation
Source	T4	
Luo	T5	
Xi	T7	
Alarm	Cv5 (Cv7, Cv12, Cv17)	
Associated	B22	

CHAPTER XII

GALL BLADDER

Traditional Chinese and Western Scientific Conceptions

The Gall-Bladder is a True and Upright Official: it Controls Judgements

'*The gall-bladder is the true and upright official who excels in making decisions.*'

(Su Wen, linglan midian lun)

'*All the other eleven Zang and Fu make their decisions in the gall-bladder.*'

(Su Wen, liujie zangxiang lun)

Case History. A man in his forties was unable to decide what he wanted to do, which country abroad he wished to visit for a holiday, which car he wanted to buy, etc. He was not like a spoilt child, though this could be suggested by the above symptoms. He had a few other gall-bladder/liver symptoms, such as weakness of the muscles and the inability to eat many of the richer foods.

Pulse diagnosis showed an under-activity of gall-bladder and liver. He was about half cured of all his mental and physical symptoms after a long course of treatment, involving the use of gall-bladder and liver points.

The Gall-Bladder is the Fu of Internal Purity

'*The gall-bladder is a true and upright official; it stores pure and clean fluid, therefore it is called the Fu of internal purity. That with which all the other Fu are filled is impure, and only the gall-bladder is filled with the pure.*'

(Zhangshi leijing)

Although the gall-bladder is one of the Fu, it is different from the rest. The other Fu either store or transport impure matter such as water and nourishment, faeces and urine; only the gall-bladder fluid, bile, is not impure.

The Reciprocal Relationship between the Liver and the Gall-Bladder

The ability to make plans and judgements is not only decided by the strength or weakness of the gall-bladder Qi, but is also connected with the liver, because the liver and gall-bladder are mutually exterior and interior.

'*The gall-bladder is appended to the liver and they help one another. Even if the liver Qi is strong, without the gall-bladder there is no decision If the liver and gall-bladder mutually assist, bravery and courage are then created.*'

(Zhangshi leijing)

Thus the idea that the liver controls planning and the gall-bladder controls deciding have a mutual connection. This may be seen clinically in those whose gall-bladder fire is vigorous and abundant, where there are often the symptoms of liver Yang partially violent, in which case the patient becomes agitated and easily enraged. If the gall-bladder Qi is deficient there is often a partial decaying of liver Qi and these patients are often timid and reluctant to speak. In treating these cases, liver-balancing medicine will usually sedate the spleen fire; and spleen-fire sedating medicine will usually balance the liver.

The exterior-interior relationship of the gall-bladder and liver is more intimate than that of other coupled organs so that at times it is impossible to distinguish between one and the other. Perhaps some of the functions ascribed to the liver should be classified under the gall-bladder and vice versa. For this reason both sections should be read together.

Case History. A man told me that his wife had been bad tempered, brooding and moody for a few years, and that the slightest thing would cause her to explode in an outburst of temper. Previously she had been quite different—it was as if she were now a different person. The lady in question was quite willing to be treated, for she had herself noticed that her personality had become changed, against her own wish, and she did not like being bad tempered. She felt there was something wrong which she could not control with her own will power.

Pulse diagnosis showed an over-activity of the liver and gall-bladder. Her face, forehead and neck, were slightly purple, as may sometimes be noticed in this condition. She was markedly better from the first treatment (Liv8 and G40), to the delight of her husband, children and herself.

She was cured in three treatments. To keep everything in check, I saw her for one treatment at half-yearly intervals afterwards.

Symptomatology

Main Meridian Symptoms

Bitter taste in mouth, deafness, frequent sighing, aching chest and ribs, inability to turn body easily, skin becoming pasty coloured, pain in temples, pain below jaws, pain in outer corner of eye, swelling of supra-clavicular fossa, swelling in front of neck, redness and swelling under armpits, pain under ribs, perspiration comes for no reason, pain or loss of function along course of meridian.

SYMPTOMS OF EXCESS

Limbs slightly cold, ? stupor.

SYMPTOMS OF INSUFFICIENCY

Weakness of the legs, difficulty in standing once seated.

Gall-Bladder Cold Symptoms

The gall-bladder has the function of purifying the Yang; if pure Yang cannot spread this can give rise to symptoms in the chest and stomach, a troubled feeling and melancholy, dizziness in the head and vomiting, insomnia, tongue furred slippery and greasy. The reasons for this are that pure Yang does not ascend and turbid phlegm is not transformed.

Gall-Bladder Hot Symptoms

Bitter mouth and proneness to anger, clear bitter fluid suddenly appears in mouth from the stomach, possibly alternating cold and heat, restless sleep at night, pulse wiry and rapid. At the same time there is often foggy vision, deafness, ribs are painful. The bitter mouth symptom is usually caused by liver heat influencing the gall-bladder. If gall-bladder heat includes damp this can cause yellow jaundice, and if severe, troubled heart and nervousness, inability to sit or lie down peacefully.

Gall-Bladder Empty Symptoms

The causes of gall-bladder empty and liver empty are basically the same, both being concerned with blood empty and deficient. Thus both liver and gall-bladder empty have the symptoms of dizziness of the head, susceptibility to fright, blurred vision. However gall-bladder empty also has the important symptom of insomnia, cowardliness, timidity, fondness of sighing.

Gall-Bladder Full Symptoms

If the gall-bladder is full then it is easy to become angry, the chest feels full and melancholy, and there may be swelling and pain below ribs. If the condition is severe then there may be pain and inability to turn the body, face coloured like dust, dry skin, fondess for sleep, and pain in sides of head, forehead and corners of eyes.

The pulse is wiry and full.

Connecting Meridian (Luo) Symptoms

SYMPTOMS OF EXCESS

Cold in extremities.

SYMPTOMS OF INSUFFICIENCY

Legs weak, and inability to walk, or to rise after sitting down.

Muscle Meridian Symptoms

Muscular cramp of the fourth toe, of the outer side of the knee, the knee cannot be bent, cramp in the muscles at the back of the knee. Muscular pain at front and side of thigh, buttocks and anal region, lateral side of the abdomen and thorax, lateral side of the neck and face.

The left and right sides of the meridian are linked via the summit of the cranium and also partly follow the course of the Yin and Yang qiao mo, hence if there is an injury to the left temple there may be paralysis of the right leg.

Course of Meridians

Lung Main Meridian

Principal Course

The meridian starts at the outer corner of the eye at G1, zig-zags over the side of the head, goes down the lateral side of the body and embryologically posterior (external) surface of the leg, between the other two Yang meridians, to end at the fourth toe at G44.

Special Details

The meridian starts at the outer corner of the eye at G1 and then covers a zig-zag course over the side of the head and neck to G21.

From G21 the meridian goes over the shoulder to Gv14, B11, (?T15), Si12 to S12.

From S12 to G22, G23 (? via Cx1 and Liv14) to G24 and thence down the side of the abdomen to G29.

From G29 over the sacrum to B31, B33, Gv1 to G30.

From G30, down the outside of the leg to G44.

Sometimes the position of G35 and G36 are reversed.

A branch from G1 goes to S8, Si18, S3 to S12 where it meets the main meridian. The branch then continues over the chest to G24 (possibly Cx1 and Liv14 are on this branch).

From G24 the branch continues over the abdomen via Liv13 (or possibly Liv13 is on the main meridian between G24 and G25) to S30 and thence joins the main meridian at G30.

A branch leaves G20, goes to T17, penetrates the ear to emerge at Si19 (with possibly a continuation to S2 and thence T22).

From G7 a branch goes to T20 (or possibly T20 lies on the main meridian between G7 and G8).

A branch goes from G14 to B1.

(? From G3 to S1 to G4.)

A branch goes from G41 to Liv1.

Gall Bladder connecting Meridian (Luo)—G37

The meridian begins above the external malleolus at G37, and descends to the dorsum of the foot. It links with the liver meridian Luo.

Gall-Bladder Muscle Meridian

The meridian begins on the lateral side of the end of the fourth toe, unites at the external malleolus; ascends the lower leg and unites at the lateral side of the knee. Another part of the meridian continues up the lateral side of the leg and unites on the anterior surface of the thigh at S32. The main meridian muscle continues upwards and sends a branch to unite at the anus. It continues over the lateral side of the body and front of the shoulder joint to unite at the supra-clavicular fossa. A separate course runs anteriorly to link with the breast. The main meridian muscle ascends behind the ear to the top of the cranium where it meets the division from the other side of the body; it descends at the side of the jaw, and then ascends to unite at the side of the nose. A branch ascends to unite at the outer corner of the eye.

Gall-Bladder and Liver Divergent Meridians

Gall-Bladder Divergent Meridian

The gall-bladder divergent meridian leaves the gall-bladder main meridian at the buttocks, which it encircles, to enter the pubic area, where it meets the liver meridian. The divergence ascends to the lower border of the ribs whence it enters the gall bladder, to which it belongs, and disperses in the liver. It ascends to penetrate the heart and thence goes along the side of the neck, jaw and cheek, to the outer corner of the eye where it meets the main gall-bladder meridian.

Liver Divergent Meridian

The liver divergent meridian leaves the main liver meridian on the dorsum of the foot; it ascends up the inside of the leg to the pubic area where it meets the gall-bladder divergent meridian, whose course it then follows to the outer corner of the eye.

Important Points

Metal	G44	
Water	G43	Tonification
Wood	G41	Wood point of Yang wood meridian
Fire	G38	Sedation
Earth	G34	
Source	G40	
Luo	G37	
Xi	G36	
Alarm	G24	
Associated	B19	

CHAPTER XIII

LIVER

Traditional Chinese and Western Scientific Conceptions

The Storing of Blood by the Liver

'*The liver stores blood.*'

(Ling Shu, bian shen pian)

'*Thus when men lie down the blood returns to the liver.*'

(Su Wen, wuzang shengcheng lun)

Wang Bing's commentary to the above says 'When man moves the blood travels to several meridians; when man is still the blood returns to the liver Zang.'

These extracts explain that the liver has the function of storing the blood and regulating the amount of blood. Clinically, vomiting of blood may be caused by violent anger, and can be cured by treating the liver; the theory is expressed as 'anger injures the liver', and 'the liver stores blood'. At a time of great anger the Jing Shen receives a violent stimulus and this affects the normal functioning of the liver, causing the liver Qi to rebel upwards, so that it cannot maintain the function of storing the blood; the blood then rises with the Qi and flows out of the body. Thus the liver must be balanced before this complaint can be cured.

'The storing of blood by the liver,' probably refers to the portal circulation, which acts as a blood reservoir as outlined in the above three quotations. In dogs there is even an involuntary sphincter muscle at the junction of the hepatic vein and the inferior vena cava. Haemoptysis may be the result of oesophageal varices consequent on portal obstruction.

Haemorrhoids are at least partially associated with the liver, presumably because the portal circulation passes through the liver. Patients who have had mild haemorrhoids, which did not bother them so that they forgot to mention it when I treated some other condition, have frequently noticed an improvement in their haemorrhoids if I treated their liver (either because of their other condition or because of the pulse and other methods of diagnosis).

Sometimes haemorrhoids are better treated via the bladder meridian for the bladder divergent meridian passes alongside the anus. B56, B57, B58 may be used. Gv1 or other points in the sacral area may also help. Gv20, at the opposite end of the body to the anus is useful, working via the law of polarity.

Patients who bruise easily normally have a dysfunction of their liver. This is frequently the case with women who may bruise with the slightest pressure on their skin, or even spontaneously for no apparent reason. Such conditions can presumably be at least partially explained by the fact that the clotting factors in the blood, such as prothrombin, fibrinogen and heparin are manufactured in the liver. This symptom is very marked in those who are jaundiced, making surgery with adequate haemostasis difficult.

Case History. A lady bruised so easily that one had the incorrect impression her husband had maltreated her. She was improved, but not completely cured, by treating the liver.

In general, at least in my experience, this condition of bruising easily can usually be improved by treating the liver, though sometimes it may be completely cured and sometimes this treatment has no effect at all.

The Liver as the General Official and Controller of Planning

The liver has the functions of guarding against insults from outside, considering plans, and resisting disease and evils.

The detoxification of drugs takes place mostly in the liver. Hence patients who have taken many drugs, which is often the case, will have to have their livers treated in addition to whatever other disease they have. Sometimes it may be difficult to distinguish the original disease from the drug induced disease.

The Relationship between the Liver and Muscles, and Finger and Toe Nails

The muscles are controlled by the liver.

If when examining a patient there are symptoms such as aching and pain of the muscles and bones, muscular spasm and cramp, spasms of the muscles of the tongue, it may be deduced that there is disease of the liver and muscles.

The strength and thickness of the finger nails and their colour and texture are also determined by the state of health of the liver. For instance, in patients whose liver (and blood) is deficient, the finger nails are often soft and thin, the colour underneath the nails is very pale, and in some cases the nails are cracked. Moreover the nails of old people may be withered when the liver and blood are no longer flourishing.

'The liver . . . its external manifestation is in the nails.'

(Su Wen, lu chie zhan zang lun)

'Nails are the surplus of muscles.'

(Zhubing yuanhou lun)

A patient whose liver is not functioning correctly normally finds that in the morning, when he feels worst, he is only able to run slowly; in the evening when he feels better, he can run faster. Other muscular activities follow the same hepatic pattern.

The above can perhaps be supported by the fact that parenteral bile salts cause skeletal muscular hyperactivity, twitching and spasm. (Ries and Still, 1930.)

The Relationship between the Liver and the Eyes

In general, red, swollen, painful and acute eye diseases belong to the liver fire ascending group; the symptoms of mild blurred vision, photophobia, spots in front of the eyes, weak eyesight, eyes dizzy, both eyes dry or night blindness, generally belong to the 'blood not nourishing the liver' group.

In clinical practice the liver is the organ most often associated with eye diseases. The local point which has the most effect on the eye is G20—a point that is the particular speciality of Dr Li Zhi-ming of Peking.

Why the eye and liver should be related to one another, as observed in clinical experience, and as recognised in the laws of acupuncture, is not clear. Possibly melanin is a partial bridge. On the one hand melanin is produced in the liver: tyrosin→tyrosinase→ melanin; on the other hand the choroid of the eye is the only part of the body where melanin is stored in quantity. In jaundice melanin is also produced in the skin by melanoblasts.

Case History. A patient was only able to read a book for half an hour, after which his eyes were too tired to read any more. He had been to a good ophthalmologist and optician.

Pulse diagnosis showed an over-activity of the liver. He was cured in five treatments by using Liv8 and G20. He can now read for several hours at a time.

Psychology

The liver likes cheerfulness and reasonableness; anger and depression are the main causes of psychosomatic hepatic diseases.

In nearly all psychiatric diseases where depression or outbursts of anger are the leading symptom, the liver is most often the physical component of the disease. Once a psychiatric disorder has become so profound that the liver is actually affected, it would require extremely intensive psychotherapy to cure. My own experience is that the depression can more easily be cured by treating the liver.

Depression is a well-known complication of jaundice. For there to be a depression, however, it is not necessary for the hepatic damage to be of such a degree as to produce jaundice. Possibly different factors are involved from those which are invariably associated with jaundice. In German, if someone is bad tempered, one asks: 'Has a flea crawled across your liver?'

Case History. A patient was continuously depressed, took no interest in life and hardly did any work. He was cured by treating Liv6 and Liv13. At the same time he noticed that his appetite increased and that his bowel motions became darker.

The Liver and Water Retention

There are many causes of water retention, the more obvious being renal and cardiac. The liver however plays a dominant role in a certain type which is characterised by a very slight puffiness of the subcutaneous tissues, giving the skin a slightly thickened appearance. It is not a pitting oedema, nor does gravity play a role. Normally this puffiness of the skin is fairly generalised over the whole body. A localised form of this oedema occurs supraorbitally, as a puffy swelling between the eyebrows and eyelids.

Those women who gain or lose several pounds in weight during the course of a single day, or who gain more than the usual amount of weight premenstrually, usually have a dysfunction of the liver. In addition they often have premenstrual tension and depression, and this can be cured at the same time via the liver.

In a few women, the water retention is localised in the breasts, though in the reverse sense to the above example, for when there is a dysfunction of the liver the breasts become small; when the liver function has been normalised, the breasts enlarge to their normal size. There may be a difference by as much as four inches in the measurement round the bust. This association between liver and breast could be explained via the gall bladder muscle meridian, which goes to the breast.

Desoxycholic acid, one of the bile acids, exerts a mild diuretic action in patients with heart failure and oedema. (Modell & Gold, 1944.)

Case History. A patient gained four pounds whenever she did not feel well, with puffiness of the skin, supraorbital oedema, headache and spots before the eyes. She was cured by merely treating the liver at Liv8.

The Liver and Allergy

Most allergies can be cured at least partially, by treating the liver, though the treatment need not, of course, be by acupuncture; any effective method will suffice. Usually, to obtain the maximum benefit, there are additional localising factors, called target areas by Dr Richard Mackarness, and these should be treated in addition, though the liver itself will nearly always achieve the main response.

Amongst the allergies which may be treated there are:—one type of asthma, one type of hay fever, urticaria, angioneurotic oedema, the numerous food allergies, and contact dermatitis.

The milder and moderate allergies can normally be cured or considerably helped. I imagine the very severe cases, such as have anaphylactic shock from just the taste of an oyster, would be better but not cured, for their other concomitant symptoms such as migraine are undoubtedly better. I have considered it prudent however not to test them with another oyster. Contact dermatitis can, as a rule, be helped a little. Food allergies are alleviated a moderate amount, though only a few completely cured.

Case History. A patient had a rash, always on the same place on the lower leg, whenever he ate egg. Even one egg in a large cake was sufficient. Sometimes he had other allergic symptoms in addition.

After treating the liver, and to a slight extent the spleen and kidney, he was able to eat as much cake as he liked and, in addition, one egg a week, without symptoms. He was not cured for life though, and required a single booster treatment once or twice a year thereafter.

The Liver and Digestive System

Many digestive disturbances in which discomfort is felt in the upper abdomen are hepatic. There may be: swelling, discomfort, feeling of fullness, feeling as if food is lying undigested in stomach, one type of duodenal ulcer, etc. If there is insufficient bile the stools will be pale, at least intermittently. There may be spasm of the colon with ribbon stools, constipation, or a bitter taste in the mouth and a dry mouth—part of the liver meridian runs round the inside of the mouth.

Parenteral bile salts increase the motor activity of the gastro-intestinal tract.

The Liver and Life

A general sense of well-being and energy is more often dependent on the liver than any other organ in the body—at least in my experience.

Presumably this is because the liver is the centre of metabolism, which is after all the most important aspect of life. From the point of view of evolution the metabolism is what distinguishes the animate from the inanimate. Amoebae have a metabolism. Only at a later stage of evolution do supportive organs such as the heart, kidney or a nervous system, develop.

Symptomatology

Main Meridian Symptoms

Aching of waist, difficulty in looking up or down, distention of lower abdomen, dry throat, face looks as if it is covered with a layer of dust, asthma, dyspnoea, does not digest food, vomiting, diarrhoea, Qi rebels, loss of control of urination and defaecation—or no relief from these acts, depression, bad-temper, hernia.

SYMPTOMS OF EXCESS

Swelling of the penis, scrotal diseases, excessive erection.

SYMPTOMS OF INSUFFICIENCY

Pruritus.

Traditional Classification

The mother of liver wood is kidney water, and if kidney water is deficient it easily causes liver Yang violent diseases, and this is called 'water does not submerge wood'.

Among liver disease symptoms, the most prominent is a type which belongs to wind (inner wind, not the wind of the six excesses).

If, for example, there is dizziness, spasms, convulsions etc., it is what the Su Wen describes as 'all wind, collapsing and dizziness belong to the liver'.

Liver Cold Symptoms

The symptoms of liver cold generally appear in the Lower Warmer; if there is cold then the muscles and vessels contract and Qi and blood are congealed and blocked. This may cause contraction of the scrotum and pain in the testicles, pain and swelling in the lower abdomen.

The pulse is generally deep and wiry, but slow.

Liver Hot Symptoms

The cause of liver hot symptoms is generally 'wood vigorous creates fire'. Among them are the localised diseases such as pain in the sides, dizziness, proneness to anger, pain in the back, spasms and convulsions, 'extreme heat creates wind'. These are similar to liver full symptoms, but there are also many heat manifestations of liver fire burning upwards, such as swelling, pain and redness of eyes, excessive lachrymation, bitter mouth, red tongue, dry mouth, troubled and hot heart, restless sleep at night, being startled and agitated during sleep. It can also move downwards and become Yin internal pain, urethral discharge, haematuria, etc.

The pulse is wiry and rapid.

Liver Empty Symptoms

These generally arise from blood fluid being decayed and small in quantity, or from deficiency of kidney water and inability to submerge wood. The principle symptoms are tinnitus, dizziness, eyes dry, partial blindness.

The pulse is usually wiry, fine but weak.

If the liver is empty and there is little blood, it cannot nourish the muscles and vessels, so spasms and convulsions occur; possibly limbs and body numb, nails dried up and blue-green, desire to lie down. The cause of this is Yin empty, Yang vigorous, Yin and Yang are not of the same strength.

Liver Full Symptoms

If the liver Qi is excessive it causes people easily to become angry, Qi and blood are depressed and congealed, the chest is distended and painful and this distension and pain may extend to the abdomen, liver Qi rebels horizontally and may invade the stomach and spleen causing pain in the stomach and abdomen, vomiting sour-clear fluid, possibly painful diarrhoea. These are 'liver wood insulting earth'.

There is also liver Qi rebelling upwards and producing Qi blocked, dyspnoea and coughing, with haematemesis and haemoptysis in severe cases. If, in addition, there is movement of liver wind, then there can be spasms of arms and legs, rigidity, pain in the back.

The pulse is usually wiry and unyielding.

Connecting Meridian (Luo) Symptoms

SYMPTOMS OF EXCESS

Excessive erections, swelling of testicles.

SYMPTOMS OF INSUFFICIENCY

Genitalia itch violently.

Muscle Meridian Symptoms

Pain and muscular spasm along the course of the muscle meridian.

If there has been excessive sexual intercourse then there is impotence with inability to obtain an erection. If the patient suffers from cold then the penis shrivels in an inward direction; if the patient suffers from heat then the penis becomes relaxed and cannot tense.

Course of Meridians

Liver Main Meridian

Principal Course

The liver meridian originates on the big toe at Liv1. Thence it goes up the embryologically anterior surface of the leg, mostly between the other Yin meridians, then over the abdomen to end on the lower costal margin at Liv14.

Special Details

The meridian starts at the end of the big toe at Liv1, goes to Liv4, and then via Sp6 to Liv5, and thence up the leg to Liv11.

From Livɪɪ the meridian goes via Spɪ2 and Spɪ3 to Livɪ2.

From Livɪ2 the meridian loops around the genitalia going to Cv2, Cv3, Cv4 to Livɪ3, then on to Livɪ4.

From Livɪ3 it goes alongside the stomach (? going to Cvɪ2), enters the liver, to which it belongs, and connects with the gall-bladder.

From Livɪ4 the meridian passes through the diaphragm, and is then scattered through the chest and ribs, going up the back of the throat, ascending through the jaw and cheek-bones to enter the eye.

From the eye the meridian goes over the forehead to the top of the head (? Gv20).

A branch leaves the eye, descends through the lower jaw and circles round the mouth inside the lips.

Another branch leaves Livɪ4, penetrates the diaphragm, pours into the lungs and joins the meridian of the lung (Lɪ).

Liver Connecting Meridian (Luo)—Livɪ5

The meridian begins above the ankle at Livɪ5 and goes up the leg to the testicles and penis. It links with the gall-bladder meridian Luo.

Liver Muscle Meridian

The meridian begins at the big toe, unites in front of the internal malleolus; ascends along the tibia and unites at the inner side of the knee; ascends the thigh and unites at the genitalia and there collects with all the other meridian muscles.

Important Points

Wood	Livɪ	Wood point of Yin wood meridian
Fire	Liv2	Sedation
Earth	Liv3	
Metal	Liv4	
Water	Liv8	Tonification
Source	Liv3	
Luo	Liv5	
Xi	Liv6	
Alarm	Livɪ4	
Associated	Bɪ8	

CHAPTER XIV

EIGHT EXTRA MERIDIANS

(also Conception and Governing Vessel Connecting Meridians)

Ren Mo

(Conception or pregnancy Vessel)

Course

Master point L7   *Coupled point* K3

The meridian arises at Cv1, going up the midline of the abdomen, thorax, neck and chin, and terminates below the lower lip at Cv24.

From Cv24 a branch goes round the lips, sending an off-shoot to S4, where it enters the eyes, thus joining the stomach and Yang qiao meridians.

Function and Symptomatology

The Ren mo is the 'sea' of the Yin meridians. The three lower Yin, the Yin qiao and Chong mo join the Ren mo. Therefore the Ren mo controls the Yin meridians of the body.

'The vessel of conception connects ↲ through way . . . therefore the menses descend at the right time' '. . . controls pregnancy nourishment.' ' . . . the root of conception in the woman.'

The vertebral column belongs to Yang, the diaphragm to Yin, the lower abdomen is the Yin within the Yin. Diseases of the Ren mo therefore affect the lower abdomen and lower warmer. 'The male contracts the seven types of herniae; the female has red and white vaginal discharge or fibroids.' 'Distress in the lower abdomen, with pain encircling the navel going to the pubic bone with sharp pain in the genitalia.' 'If the abdomen is distressed there is Qi, like a finger, ascending to attack the heart. The patient can neither bend down nor straighten up.' There may be lumbago, pain at the back of the head and neck or abscesses of the mouth and tongue.

Cv4 may be used for menstrual disturbances, vaginal discharge, herniae and lunacy.

The individual points on this meridian have an effect on those organs which are roughly on the same segmental level: The lower points genito-urinary, the middle points digestive, the upper points thoracic.

Commoner Diseases

Asthma, bronchitis, pneumonia, pleurisy, asthenia, pulmonary T.B., laryngitis, cough, rhinitis, hay fever, emphysema, haemoptysis, influenza, sneezing, coryza, whooping cough, aphonia, hot flushes, meningitis of children, convulsions or epilepsy (or Yin wei mo), eczema, diabetes, dyspepsia, pharyngitis, mouth diseases (or Du mo), alimentary intoxication, menstrual disorders—not in virgins (or Dai mo), breast abscess, pain head and neck.

Vessel of Conception Connecting Meridian (Luo)—Cv15

The meridian begins at Cv15 and descends to scatter in the abdomen.

SYMPTOMS OF EXCESS

Skin of abdomen painful.

SYMPTOMS OF INSUFFICIENCY

Skin of abdomen itches.

Du Mo
(*Governing Vessel*)

Course

Master point Si3   *Coupled point* B62

The governing vessel begins at the tip of the coccyx at Gv1, sending a branch forward on the perineum to Cv1. The meridian continues up the spines of the vertebrae, at the same time uniting with them. At Gv16, below the occiput, it enters the brain, to reach the top of the head. It descends over the forehead and nose, to curl around the upper lip, and ends on the gum between the incisor teeth at Gv28.

A branch goes from Gv12, via B12 on both sides, to Gv13.

There are some additional points, apart from the 28 numbered points, on this meridian.

This meridian joins the Ren mo by sending a branch from Gv28 to Cv24, and also joins the stomach meridian.

Function and Symptomatology

The governing vessel unites the Yang Qi of the whole body. The three Yang meridians of the arms and the three Yang meridians of the legs join the Du mo, the most Yang of all the Yang meridians.

The constitution is partly dependent on the Du mo, for it is connected with the kidney. From Cv1 it ascends to the right kidney (fire), whereby Yin pertains to Yang. From XH3 (Tai Yang = Supreme Yang or the sun) it descends (? governing vessel connecting meridian) to the left kidney (water), whereby Yang pertains to Yin.

When the meridian is overactive, the spine becomes stiff, as the meridian Qi is blocked; there is also headache and pain in the eyes. When underactive, the head feels heavy, and the patient walks with rounded shoulders, as the pure Yang Qi is unable to rise.

In disease the Du mo unifies the Yang Qi of the whole body and unites with the Yin Qi, thus not only will there be stiffening of the spine at the waist but also 'insanity in adults and convulsions in children'. The above may also be due to the Du mo going to the brain. It may be treated via Gv20.

As the Du mo originates in the perineum, it may be associated with haemorrhoids, retention of urine, herniae and sterility.

The individual points on this meridian have an effect on the same organ as the associated points on the same level: e.g. Gv4 is on the same level as B23, both having an effect on the kidney; and Gv12 is on the same level as B13, both having an effect on the lung.

All points in the lumbo-sacral region, whether they be on the governing vessel or the bladder meridian, have an effect on the kidney/bladder in addition to whatever other effect they may have.

Commoner Diseases

Headache (or Yang wei mo), pain in neck and back especially in the region of vertebra C7, neuralgia of forehead and eyebrows, lumbago, warm back, contraction of throat jaw and neck, torticollis, conjunctivitis, running eyes, over stimulation, hallucinations, dementia, epilepsy, vertigo, toothache (or Yang wei mo), tonsillitis, productive cough, mouth diseases (or Ren mo), deafness, cold extremities.

Governing Vessel Connecting Meridian (Luo)—Gv1

The meridian begins at Gv1, ascends paravertebrably to the nape of the neck, disperses over the occiput, descends and when it reaches the shoulders links with the bladder connecting meridian. It penetrates to pass through the inside of the spine.

SYMPTOMS OF EXCESS

Spine stiff and straight, cannot easily bend.

SYMPTOMS OF INSUFFICIENCY

Head heavy and shaking.

Chong Mo
(*Penetrating vessel*)

Course

Master point Sp4   *Coupled point* Cx6

This meridian together with the Ren mo arises in the uterus, represented by Cv1. It ascends the coccyx, sacrum and lower lumbar spine, where it acts as the 'sea' of the Jing and Luo. The superficial part goes over the groin at S30 and then up the kidney meridian from K11 to K21, there being a branch from K15 to Cv7. Thereafter it goes over the thorax and throat to encircle the mouth.

Function and Symptomatology

The Chong mo is called 'the sea of the twelve meridians' and 'the sea of blood'. In its upward course it connects all the Yang meridians, in its downward course all the Yin meridians.

The Chong mo is initially connected with the kidney and stomach meridians: the former regulating prenatal, the latter postnatal development. It is therefore said to store the True Qi.

'It restrains and regulates the sinews and meridians of the whole body.' 'Master of diseases of the heart, the abdomen and the five Zang.'

'Qi rebels upwards from the lower abdomen, abdomen swollen and extremely painful.' 'Pain in lower abdomen ascending to seize the heart.'

The Ren mo, Du mo and Chong mo all arise at Cv1, which is connected with the uterus. The Ren mo is the sea of the Yin meridians; the Du mo the sea of the Yang meridians; the Chong mo the sea of blood. 'When the Chong mo flourishes menstruation occurs at the right time.' 'When it is not regulated miscarriage occurs, (referring in one text to the Chong mo, and in another to Chong and Ren mo).'

'In a woman the Ren and Chong mo do not unite round the lips: hence she has no beard.' 'The Chong mo originates in the genitalia and goes round the lips. In a eunuch it is cut: hence he has no beard.'

Commoner Diseases

Digestive troubles in general, aerocolon, anorexia, hiccoughs, atonic gastritis, cholecystitis, atonic constipation, difficult digestion, 'tummy ache', hyperacidity, gastric ulcer, jaundice, vomiting, bradycardia, endo or myocarditis, palpitations, lumbago (or Yang qiao mo), malaria.

Dai Mo
(Girdle vessel)

Course

Master point G41   *Coupled point* T5
The meridian encircles the body at the level of the waist—G28, G27, G26 and possibly Liv13.

Function and Symptomatology

The girdle vessel binds all the meridians that course up and down the body. If it is in disorder the abdomen is bloated or there is 'sagging of the waist as when one is seated in water.' There may be aching and pain at the level of the waist.

Menstruation may be irregular, with red or white vaginal discharge. 'All the meridians go up and down creating heat between themselves and the Dai mo. Heat and cold contend with one another, white matter becomes over-full and leaks down in a constant stream.'

Commoner Diseases

Amenorrhoea, dysmenorrhoea, menstrual disturbance—not in virgins (or Ren mo), anaemia, weakness and general fatigue, fainting, trembling, pruritus (or Yang wei mo), contracture of hands and feet, pain in arm and shoulder, pain in knee, arthritis in general, pain in leg or foot or ankle, redness of wrists and ankles, articular rheumatism (or Yang qiao mo), spasms, abdominal pain (or Ren mo), lumbago, abdominal distension, vomiting (or Chong mo), inflammation of breasts, ovaritis, thinness.

Yin Qiao Mo
(*Yin heel vessel*)

Course

Master point K3   *Coupled point* B62

The meridian begins on the medial side of the foot near K2, goes to K3, K8 and up the leg, abdomen and thorax, to the supra-clavicular fossa near S12. Thence it goes in front of S9, to the medial corner of the eye at B1, where it meets the bladder, small intestine, stomach and Yang qiao meridians.

Function and Symptomatology

See section of Yang qiao mo.

Yang Qiao Mo
(*Yang heel vessel*)

Course

Master point B62   *Coupled point* K3

The meridian begins near the external malleolus at B62, then goes to B61, B59, up the leg to G29, over the lateral side of the body to Si10, Li15, Li16, over the neck and face via S7, S6, S4 to end at B1. An extension probably goes over the cranium to G20.

Function and Symptomatology of Yin and Yang Qiao Mo

These meridians are concerned with fluid, via their kidney and bladder master points (K3 and B62), therefore 'when the Qi has a free circulation the eye is moistened, and when the Qi is not in order, the eye is not in accord'.

'When the Yang Qi is over-full and glaring, "angry eyes" result; and when the Yin Qi is over-full then the vision is blurred.' 'If there is an excess of Yang, the eyes cannot be closed; if there is an excess of Yin, the eyes are always closed.' There may also be pain at the medial corner of the eye.

'When the Yang qiao sickens, the Yin relaxes and the Yang tenses. When the Yin qiao sickens, the Yang relaxes and the Yin tenses.' According to this sickness tenses and health relaxes. 'When the Yin qiao mo tenses, the medial side of the ankle and lower leg tenses, and the lateral side of the ankle and lower leg relaxes. When the Yang qiao mo tenses, the lateral side of the ankle and lower leg tenses, and the medial side of the ankle and lower leg relaxes.'

The above tension and relaxation occurs mostly in epilepsy and other types of convulsions in which there is muscle spasm. 'If the cause is not known treat K3 in females, B62 in males.' 'If epilepsy occurs during the day treat B62, during the night K3.'

Since the Yang qiao mo is connected to the bladder meridian, there may be lumbago. Since the Yin qiao mo is connected to the kidney meridian, there may be lower abdominal pain, backache, pain in the genitalia, herniae in men and abortions in women.

'When the Yang Qi is deficient, Yin Qi is abundant, and one is often very sleepy. When the Yin Qi is deficient, Yang Qi is abundant and there is often insomnia.'

Commoner Diseases (Yin qiao mo)

Absence of sexual pleasure, impotence, frigidity, sterility, habitual abortion, difficult delivery, post-partum pains, post-partum haemorrhages, toxic pregnancy, leukorrhea, metritis, metropathia, dysmenorrhoea of virgins, ovaritis, prostatitis, seminal loss, orchitis, albuminuria, anuria, cystitis, haematuria, nephritis, enuresis, urinary retention, bladder spasm or irritation or weakness, somnolence, constipation in women, pulmonary tuberculosis, oedema in general, weakness of women and the old.

Commoner Diseases (Yang qiao mo)

Cerebral congestion, apoplexy, hemiplegia, monoplegia, para-plegia, aphasia, contractures or cramps in general, facial paralysis, lumbago (or Chong mo), sciatica, torticollis (or Ren mo), articular rheumatism (or Dai mo), articular pains (or Yang wei mo), furunculosis (or Yang wei mo), obsessions.

· Yin Wei Mo
(Yin linking vessel)

Course

Master point Cx6   *Coupled point* So4

The meridian starts on the medial side of the lower leg at K9, ascending the thigh and abdomen—Sp13, Sp15, Sp16, Liv14, and then over the chest to Cv22, to end at the larynx at Cv23.

Function and Symptomatology

'The Yin and Yang wei mo act as the binding network of all the vessels.' 'The Yin wei mo originates in the interchange of all the Yin.'

The meridian has interconnections with the Yin meridians, particularly the vessel of conception, heart and lung. 'When the Yin wei mo is diseased, the patient suffers from heart pains.' 'Yin wei mo moves all the Yin and controls Ying, Ying becomes blood, blood belongs to the heart, thus the heart is painful.' 'When the Yin wei mo is empty, the waist aches and there are pains in the genitalia'.

Commoner Diseases

Cardiac pain (or Chong mo), emotional states, unquietness, nervous laugh, failure to recall words, timidity, fear, apprehension, hypertension, mental depression, nightmares, delirium, sudden uncontrolled laughter, amnesia, agitation or epilepsy (or Ren mo), convulsions (or Ren mo), internal fullness, indigestion, abdominal pain (or Dai mo), haemorrhoids, spastic constipation, varicose veins and ulcers.

Yang Wei Mo
(*Yang linking vessel*)

Course

Master point T5   *Coupled point* G41

The meridian starts below the lateral malleolus at B63, then goes up the lateral side of the body to G35 and G24.

Then from G24 it passes behind the shoulder to Si10, T15, G21, Gv15, Gv16, G20, G19, G18, G17, G16, G15, G14 to end at G13. (The cranial course is possibly the other way round, going from G21 over the neck and side of the face to G13, and then on to G14, G15, G16, G17, G18, G19, G20, Gv16 to end at Gv15). (The part of the meridian which goes over the shoulder and neck is possibly more complex, going from G24 to Li14, T13, T15, G21, Si10, G20, Gv15, Gv16, G19 and over the cranium via the gall bladder meridian to G13.)

Function and Symptomatology

'The Yin and Yang wei mo act as the binding network of all the vessels.' 'The Yang wei mo originates at the meeting place of all the Yang.'

It has interconnections with the three Yang meridians of the legs and three Yang meridians of the arms, but most particularly with the leg greater Yang and lesser Yang—bladder and gall bladder. The former meridian controls the surface, the latter the sub-surface of the body, i.e. the protective layers of the body. Therefore 'when the Yang wei mo is diseased the patient suffers from colds and fevers.' 'Yang wei mo moves all the Yang and controls Wei, Wei becomes Qi, Qi dwells in the exterior of the body, therefore there is cold and heat.'

Commoner Diseases

Fevers in general, neuralgias in general, headache (or Du mo), pain in arms, toothache (or Du mo), pain in lower molars, pain in ears, otitis, tinnitus, arthritis of fingers and toes, articular pain (or Yang qiao mo), swelling of heel, abscess of head or mouth, furunculosis (or Yang qiao mo), acne, epistaxis, haematemesis, pruritus (or Du mo), general weakness, thinness (or Dai mo), mumps, pain and swellings of neck.

Technique for Use of Extra Meridians

1. Every extra meridian has its 'master point' and 'coupled point', as follows:

Yang/Yin: Relation I	Extra meridian	Relation II	Master	Coupled
Yang	Yang wei mo		T5	G41
	Yang qiao mo		B62	Si3
	Dai mo		G41	T5
	Du mo		Si3	B62
Yin	Yin wei mo		P6	Sp4
	Yin qiao mo		K3	L7
	Chong mo		Sp4	P6
	Ren mo		L7	K3

An extra meridian may be emptied of its excess of energy by stimulating its master point. If this has not corrected the general Yin/Yang equilibrium of the pulse, the coupled point is stimulated. If this has still not given the desired result, the midline extra meridian (Ren mo or Du mo) of the opposite sign is used. This alternative rests on the fact that the excess energy of the one sign flows into the midline extra meridian of the opposite sign.

An example. A patient is suffering from obsessions. Since in this case there is no real emotional cause for the obsession, it may be regarded as a real illness—as real as any physical illness. The symptom index shows that the Yang qiao mo is affected. This is a Yang extra meridian, and as the pulse diagnosis reveals a general excess of Yang it is perfectly legitimate to use this extra meridian. The master point B62 is bilaterally stimulated, which achieves a slight diminution of the Yang quality of the pulse, but not enough. Therefore the coupled point Si3 is stimulated, which again achieves a reduction of Yang, but not enough. Therefore the third stage is employed and the master point of the midline Yin meridian of the opposite sign is used, i.e. L7, the master point of Ren mo.

It is not usually necessary to go through all three stages of treatment as in the above example—usually the first one suffices,

2. The extra meridians may also be emptied of their excess of energy by stimulating both ends of the meridian at the same time. Either the point at the extreme end, or the penultimate point should be used.

A further guide as to deciding which extra meridian should be used is given by a consideration of the pulse as a whole. If there is a predominance of Yang, a Yang extra meridian should be used, or if there is a predominance of Yin, a Yin extra meridian should be used.

If the pulses show a predominance of Yang and the symptom index suggests a Yin extra meridian, say Ren mo, the opposite Yang meridian should be used which, in this case, would be Du mo.

Case History. A patient had suffered from hyperacidity and symptoms of gastric ulcer for six years. The symptom index suggests the use of Chong mo, which was stimulated but did not alter the symptoms. Various other procedures not involving extra meridians were also tried, but made no difference. Cognizance was then taken of the fact that the overall pulse quality was Yang, so the opposite (i.e. Yang) extra meridian was used, Dai mo. From then onwards the patient started to improve.

ILLUSTRATIONS OF THE MERIDIANS

The continuous lines represent the course of the main, connecting, muscle, divergent or extra meridians.

The finely dotted lines represent the branches, or in some instances the deeper internal course of the meridians. They also represent the connection of coupled meridians.

The heavily dotted lines represent the main meridian in the illustrations of the divergent meridians.

The broken lines represent the continuation from one drawing to another of the various meridians.

The acupuncture points on the main meridians are numbered in heavy type at a few of their representative points. Where the main meridian or its branches go to acupuncture points on other meridians, this has been indicated in all instances by lettering and numbering in lighter type. The connecting points of the connecting meridians have also been lettered and numbered in light type.

The meeting points of the muscle meridians have not been labeled.

The words alongside the illustrations, indicate the course, described in greater detail in the text of this book, of some of the meridians.

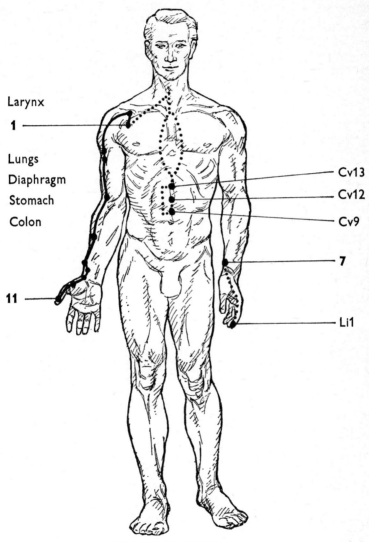

Larynx

1

Lungs
Diaphragm
Stomach
Colon

11

Cv13
Cv12
Cv9

7

Li1

LUNG MAIN MERIDIAN

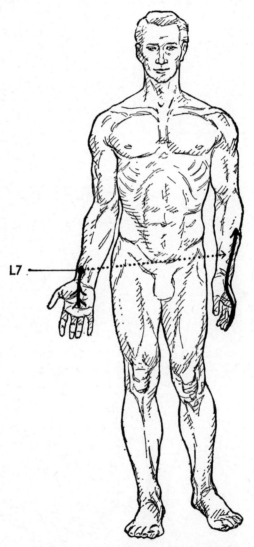

L7

LUNG CONNECTING MERIDIAN

122

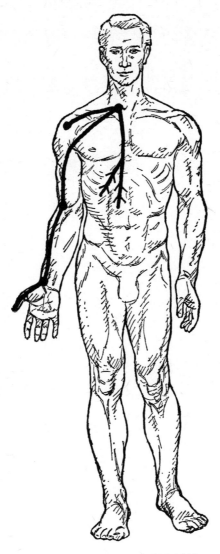

LUNG MUSCLE MERIDIAN

123

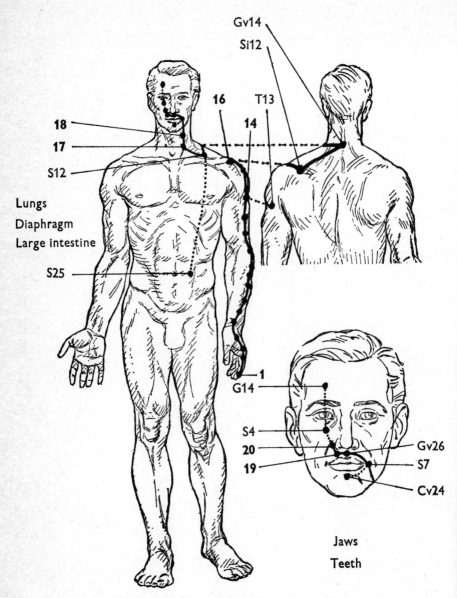

Gv14
Si12

T13

16

14

18
17
S12

Lungs
Diaphragm
Large intestine

S25

1
G14

S4

20
19

Gv26
S7
Cv24

Jaws
Teeth

LARGE INTESTINE MAIN MERIDIAN

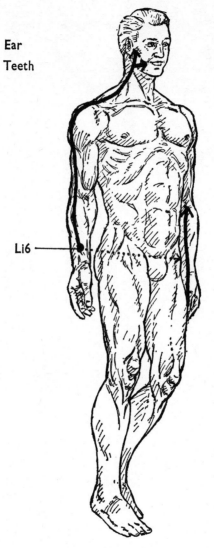

Ear
Teeth

Li6

LARGE INTESTINE CONNECTING MERIDIAN

125

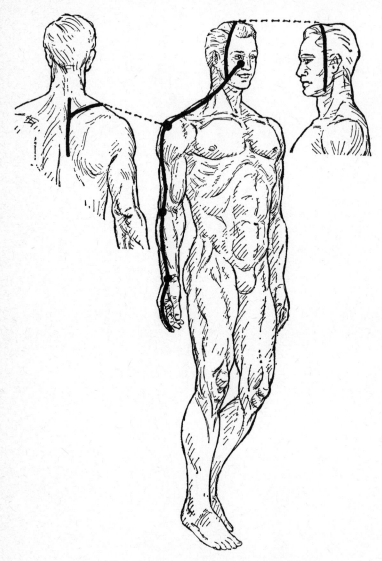

LARGE INTESTINE MUSCLE MERIDIAN

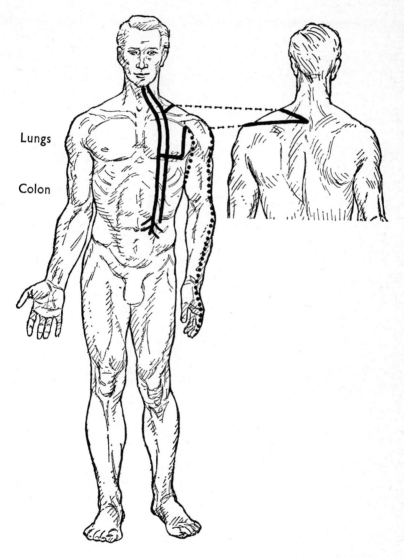

Lungs

Colon

LARGE INTESTINE AND LUNG DIVERGENT MERIDIANS

127

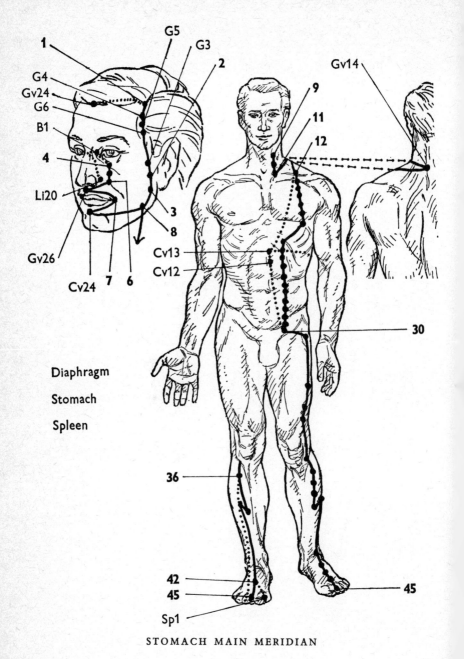

G5

1

G3

G4
Gv24
G6
B1
4
Li20
3
8
Gv26
Cv24 7 6

2

9

Gv14

11

12

30

Cv13
Cv12

36

42
45
Sp1

45

Diaphragm

Stomach

Spleen

STOMACH MAIN MERIDIAN

128

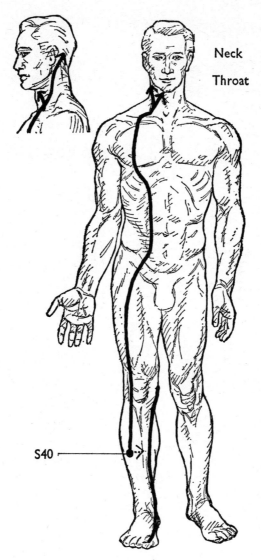

Neck

Throat

S40

STOMACH CONNECTING MERIDIAN

129

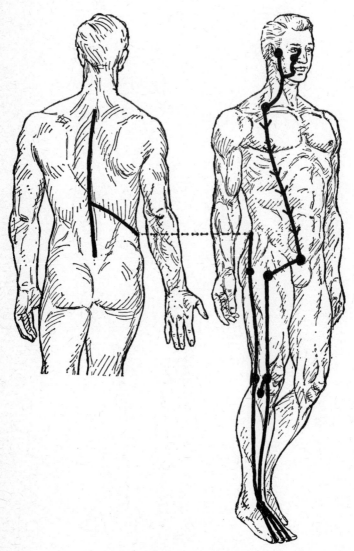

STOMACH MUSCLE MERIDIAN

130

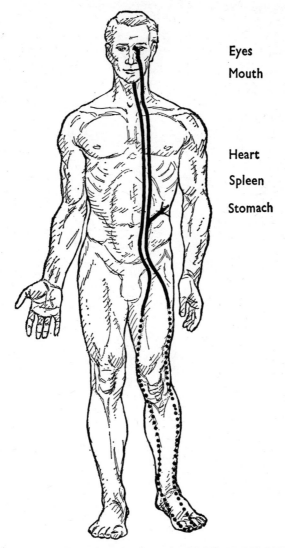

Eyes
Mouth

Heart

Spleen

Stomach

STOMACH AND SPLEEN DIVERGENT MERIDIANS

131

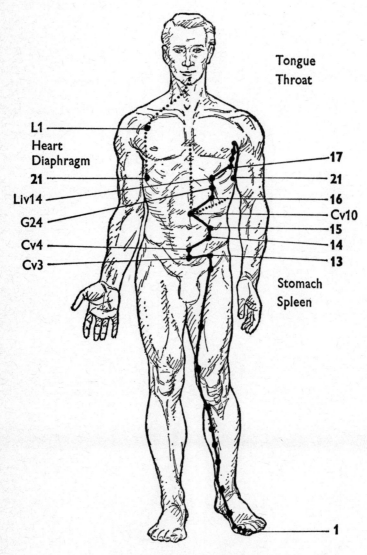

Tongue
Throat

L1

Heart
Diaphragm

21

Liv14

G24

Cv4

Cv3

17

21

16

Cv10

15

14

13

Stomach
Spleen

1

SPLEEN MAIN MERIDIAN

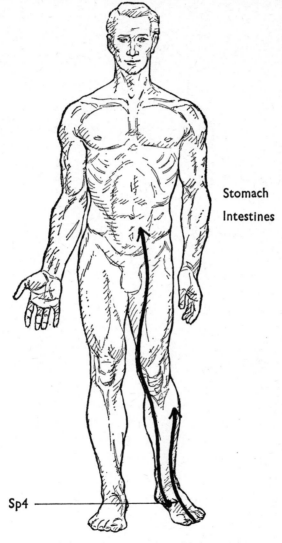

Stomach

Intestines

Sp4

SPLEEN CONNECTING MERIDIAN

133

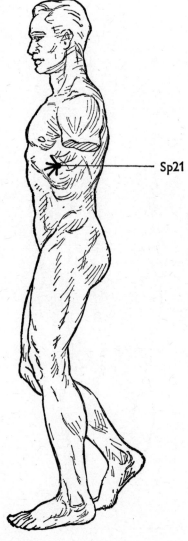

Sp21

SPLEEN GREAT CONNECTING MERIDIAN

134

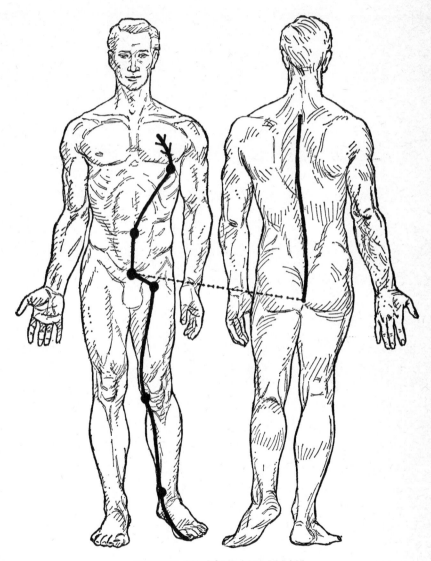

SPLEEN MUSCLE MERIDIAN

135

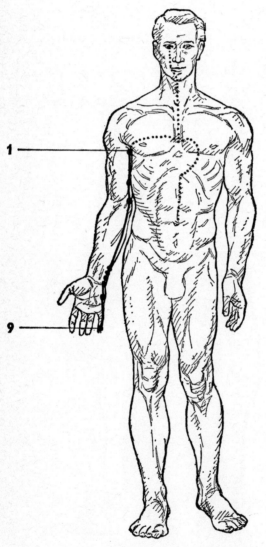

Eye

Throat

Heart
Great vessels
Diaphragm
Small intestine

HEART MAIN MERIDIAN

136

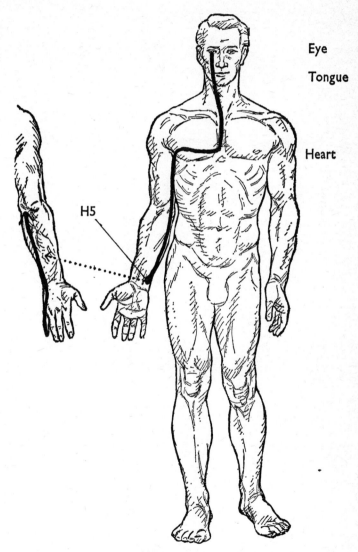

Eye

Tongue

Heart

H5

HEART CONNECTING MERIDIAN

137

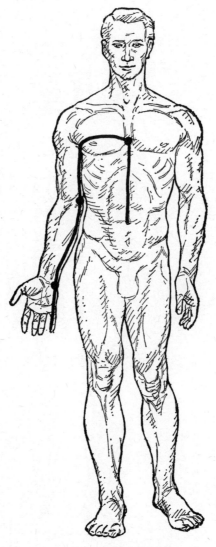

HEART MUSCLE MERIDIAN

138

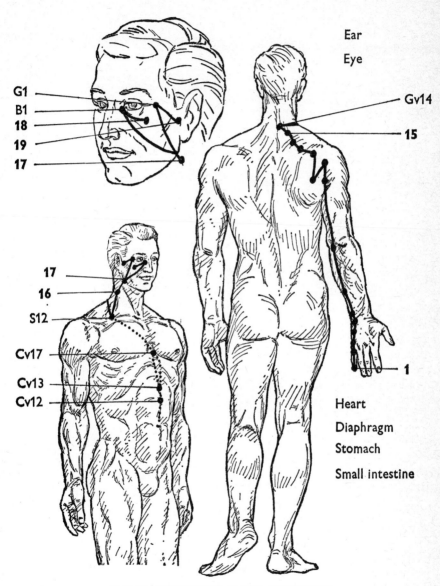

Ear
Eye

G1
B1
18
19
17

Gv14
15

17
16
S12

Cv17
Cv13
Cv12

1

Heart
Diaphragm
Stomach
Small intestine

SMALL INTESTINE MAIN MERIDIAN

139

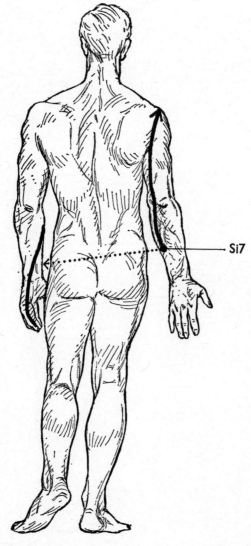

Si7

SMALL INTESTINE CONNECTING MERIDIAN

140

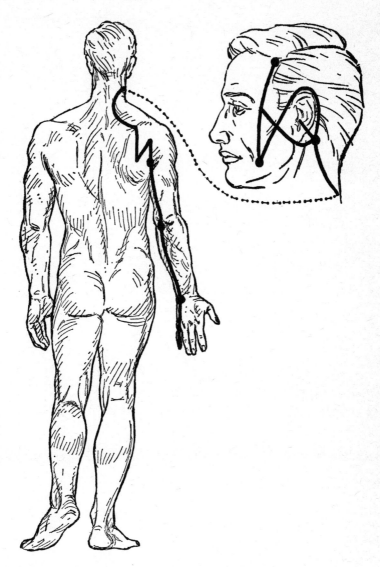

SMALL INTESTINE MUSCLE MERIDIAN

141

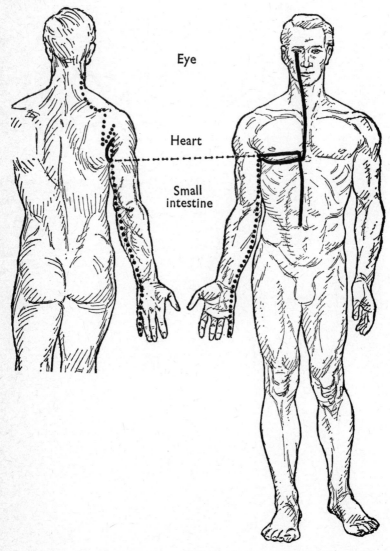

Eye

Heart

Small
intestine

SMALL INTESTINE AND HEART DIVERGENT MERIDIANS

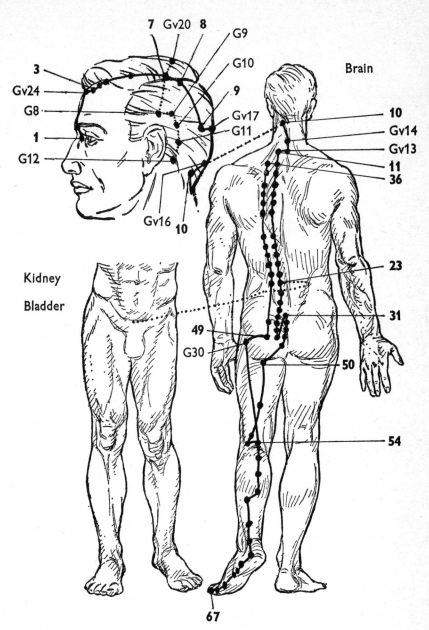

BLADDER MAIN MERIDIAN

143

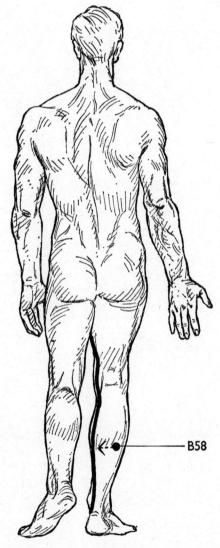

B58

BLADDER CONNECTING MERIDIAN

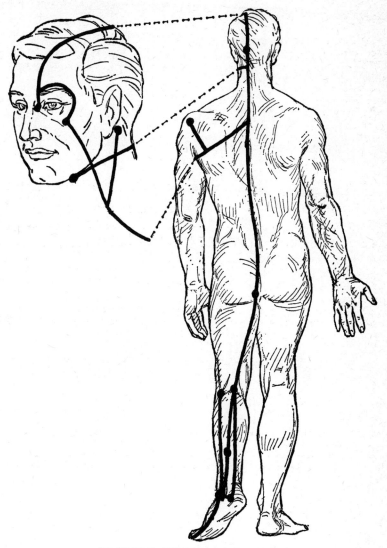

BLADDER MUSCLE MERIDIAN

145

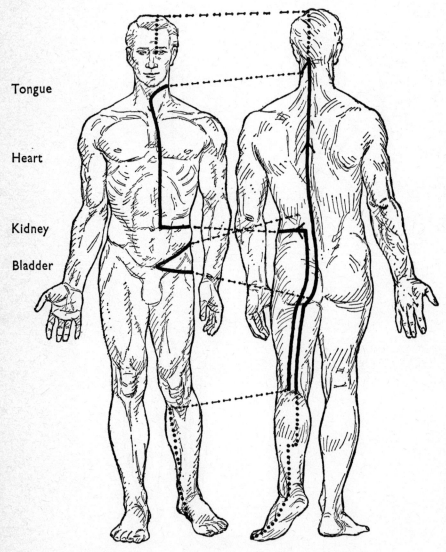

Tongue

Heart

Kidney

Bladder

BLADDER AND KIDNEY DIVERGENT MERIDIANS

146

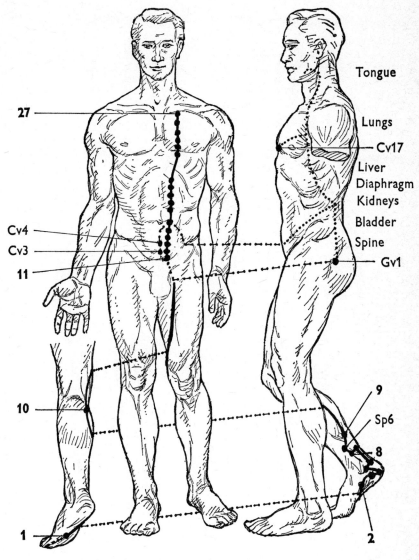

27

Cv4
Cv3
11

10

1

Tongue

Lungs

Cv17

Liver
Diaphragm
Kidneys

Bladder

Spine

Gv1

9

Sp6

8

2

KIDNEY MAIN MERIDIAN

147

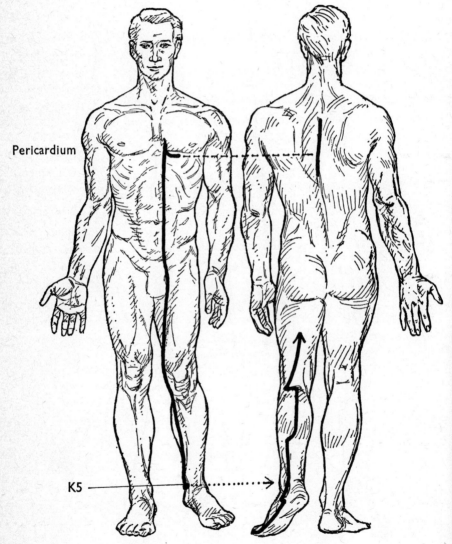

Pericardium

K5

KIDNEY CONNECTING MERIDIAN

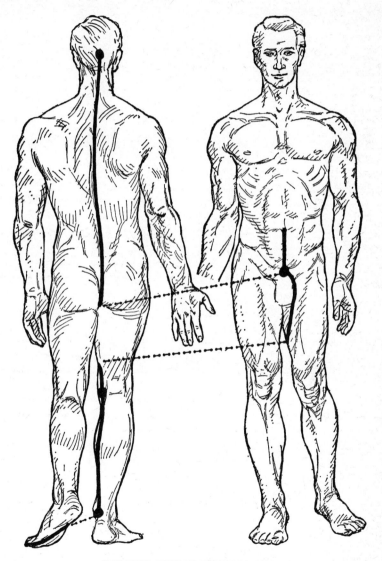

KIDNEY MUSCLE MERIDIAN

149

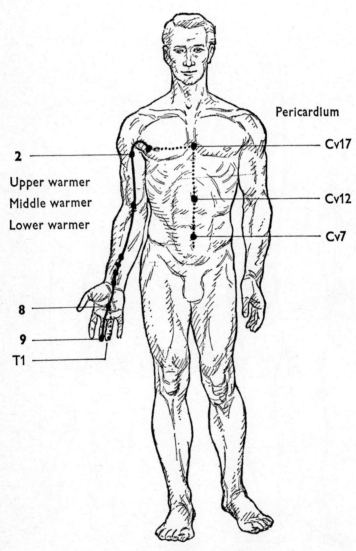

Pericardium

2

Upper warmer
Middle warmer
Lower warmer

Cv17

Cv12

Cv7

8

9

T1

CIRCULATION-SEX MAIN MERIDIAN

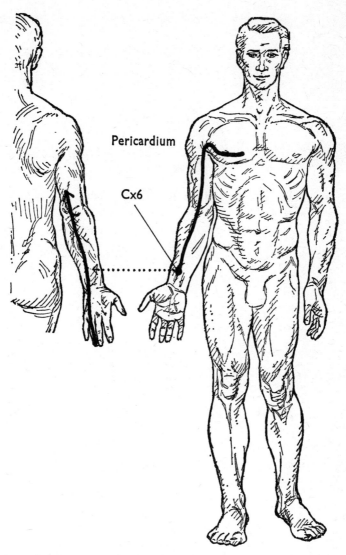

Pericardium

Cx6

CIRCULATION-SEX CONNECTING MERIDIAN

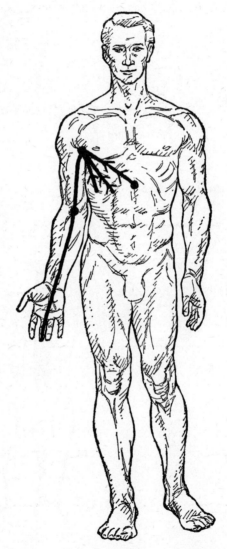

CIRCULATION-SEX MUSCLE MERIDIAN

152

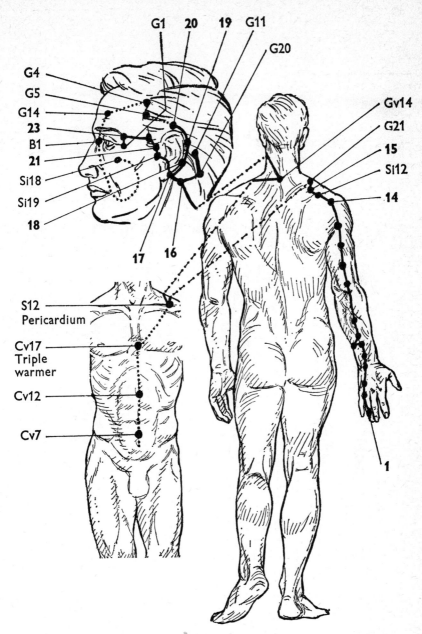

G1 20 19 G11

G20

G4
G5
G14
23
B1
21
Si18
Si19
18

17   16

Gv14
G21
15
Si12
14

S12
Pericardium

Cv17
Triple
warmer

Cv12

Cv7

1

TRIPLE WARMER MAIN MERIDIAN

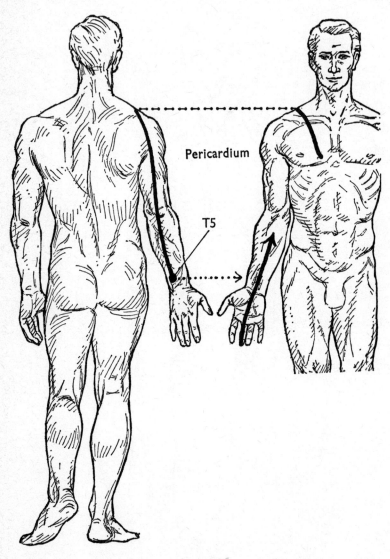

Pericardium

T5

TRIPLE WARMER CONNECTING MERIDIAN

154

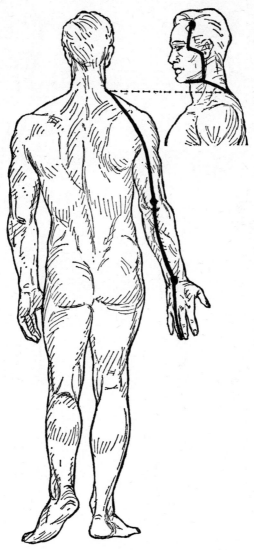

TRIPLE WARMER MUSCLE MERIDIAN

155

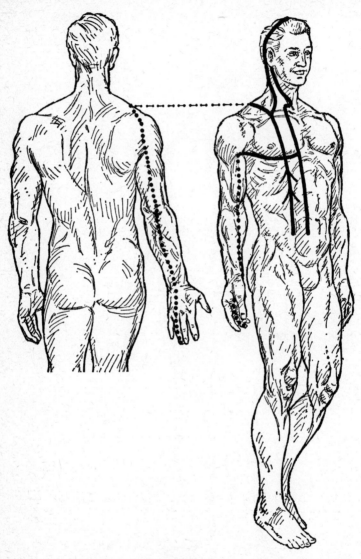

TRIPLE WARMER AND CIRCULATION-SEX DIVERGENT
MERIDIANS

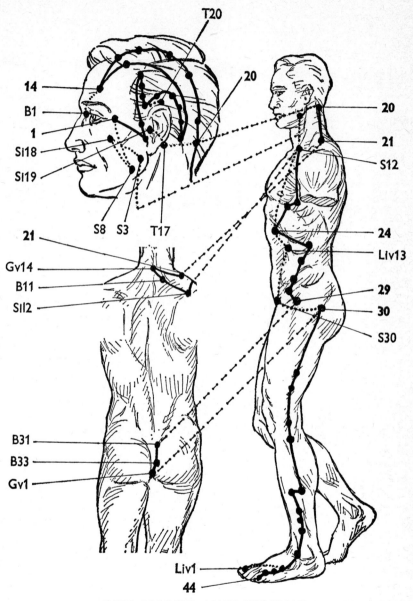

T20

20

14

B1

1

SI18

SI19

20

21

S12

S8   S3   T17

21

Gv14

B11

SII2

24

Liv13

29

30

S30

B31

B33

Gv1

Liv1

44

GALL BLADDER MAIN MERIDIAN

157

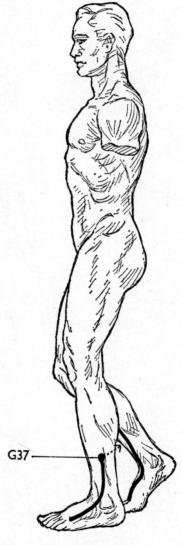

G37—

GALL BLADDER CONNECTING MERIDIAN

158

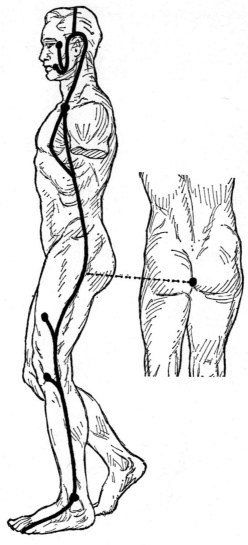

GALL BLADDER MUSCLE MERIDIAN

159

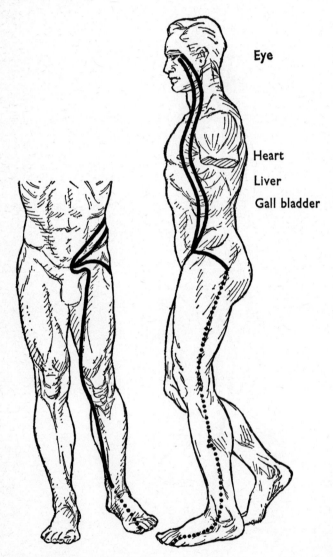

Eye

Heart

Liver

Gall bladder

GALL BLADDER AND LIVER DIVERGENT MERIDIANS

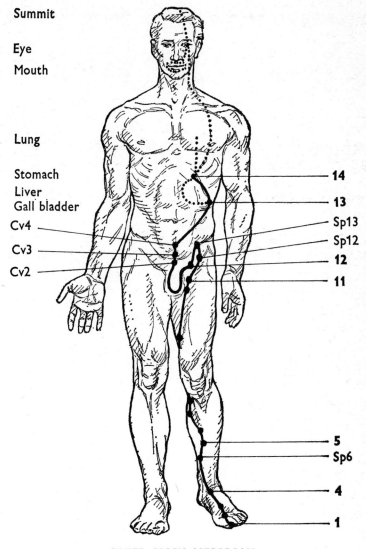

Summit

Eye
Mouth

Lung

Stomach
Liver
Gall bladder

Cv4

Cv3

Cv2

14

13

Sp13

Sp12

12

11

5

Sp6

4

1

LIVER MAIN MERIDIAN

161

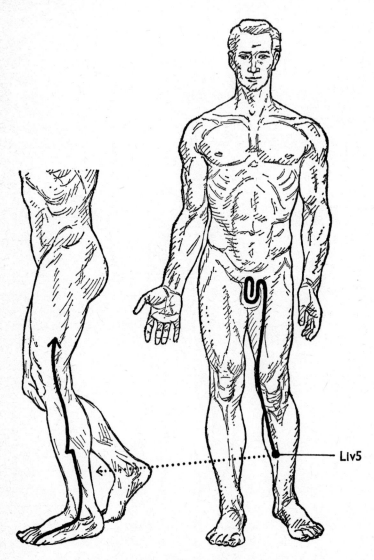

Liv5

LIVER CONNECTING MERIDIAN

162

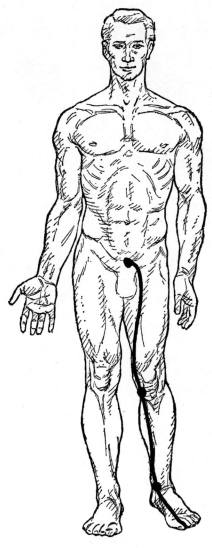

LIVER MUSCLE MERIDIAN

163

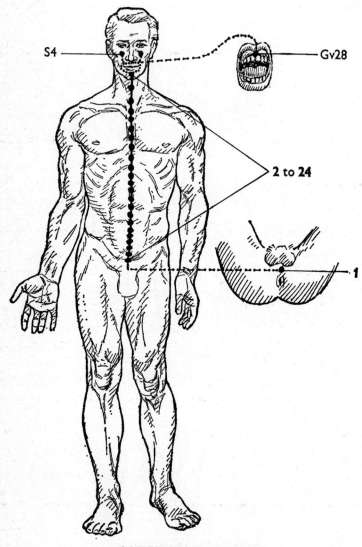

S4

Gv28

2 to 24

1

CONCEPTION VESSEL

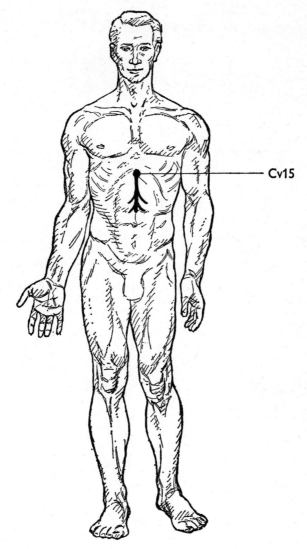

Cv15

CONCEPTION VESSEL CONNECTING MERIDIAN

165

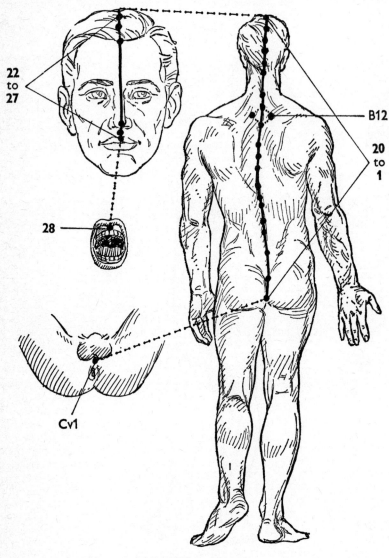

22
to
27

B12

20
to
1

28

Cv1

GOVERNING VESSEL

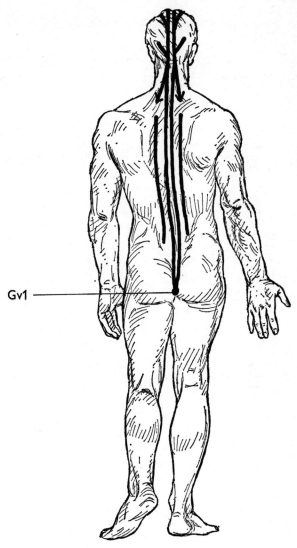

Gv1

GOVERNING VESSEL CONNECTING MERIDIAN

167

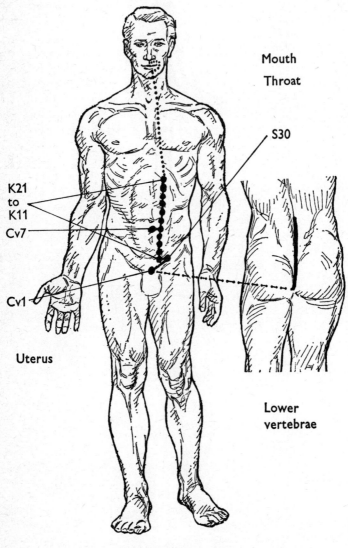

Mouth

Throat

S30

K21
to
K11

Cv7

Cv1

Uterus

Lower
vertebrae

PENETRATING VESSEL

168

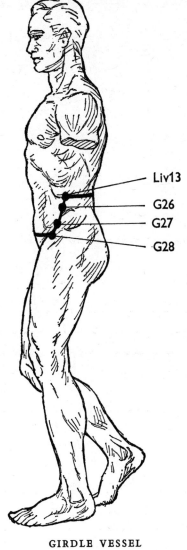

Liv13

G26

G27

G28

GIRDLE VESSEL

169

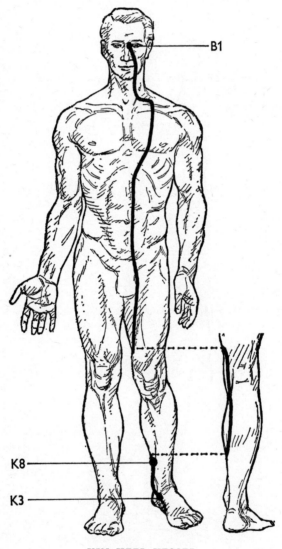

B1

K8

K3

YIN HEEL VESSEL

170

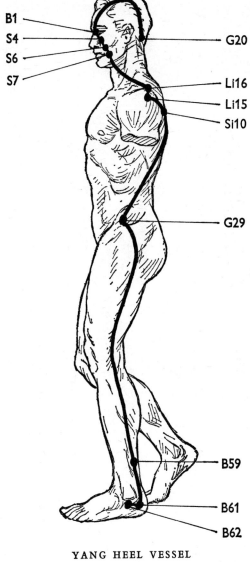

B1

S4

S6

S7

G20

Li16

Li15

Si10

G29

B59

B61

B62

YANG HEEL VESSEL

171

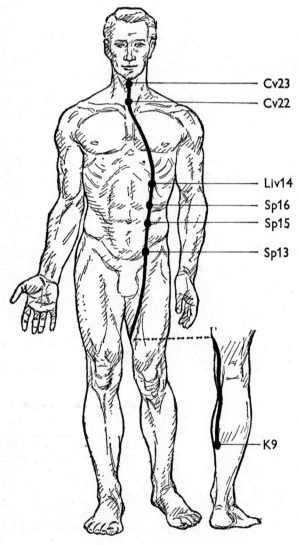

Cv23
Cv22

Liv14
Sp16
Sp15

Sp13

K9

YIN LINKING VESSEL

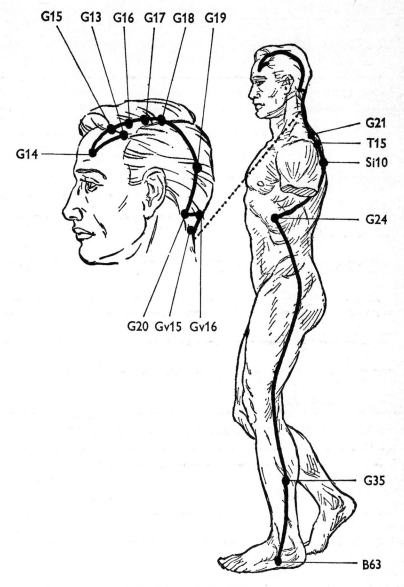

G15 G13 G16 G17 G18 G19

G14

G20 Gv15 Gv16

G21
T15
Si10

G24

G35

B63

YANG LINKING VESSEL

173

Nomenclature

Since this book was first published in 1964, there have been new editions of *Acupuncture: The Ancient Chinese Art of Healing*, *The Treatment of Disease by Acupuncture* and the *Acupuncture Charts* have been re-edited as *Atlas of Acupuncture*. In all three instances I have incorporated slight changes in nomenclature. In this reprint the 1964 nomenclature has been retained for the differences are either small or unimportant. If at a later date there is enough new material to justify a new edition, the appropriate changes will be made.

The differences are as follows:

1. The first eight points on the stomach meridian have been renumbered:

The Meridians of Acupuncture	*Acupuncture: The Ancient Chinese Art of Healing* *The Treatment of Disease by Acupuncture* *Atlas of Acupuncture* } New editions
S1	S8
S2	S7
S3	S6
S4	S1
S5	S2
S6	S3
S7	S4
S8	S5

2. The circulation-sex meridian (abbreviated Cx) is called in the 2nd edition of *Acupuncture: The Ancient Chinese Art of Healing* and in the *Atlas of Acupuncture* the pericardium meridian (abbreviated P)—as indeed it is in some parts of this book and in *The Treatment of Disease by Acupuncture*.

3. In some places the Chinese word 'lou' (or 'lo') has been translated into English—the 'connecting' meridian or point.

4. The Japanese word 'xi' has been replaced by the equivalent Chinese word 'hung', or the English 'accumulation point'.